Osteoporosis

The silent epidemic

Marilyn Glenville PhD

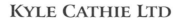

KYLE CATHIE LTD

Disclaimer
The contents of this book are for information only and are intended to assist readers in identifying symptoms and conditions they may be experiencing. This book is not intended to be a substitute for taking proper medical advice and should not be relied upon in this way. Always consult a qualified doctor or health practitioner. The author and publisher cannot accept responsibility for illness arising out of the failure to seek medical advice from a doctor.

First published in Great Britain in 2005 by
Kyle Cathie Limited
122 Arlington Road, London NW1 7HP
general.enquiries@kyle-cathie.com
www.kylecathie.com

10 9 8 7 6 5 4 3 2 1

ISBN 1 85626 607 9

Marilyn Glenville is hereby identified as the author of this work in accordance with Section 77 of the Copyright, Designs and Patents Act 1988.

Senior Editor Muna Reyal
Designer Robert Updegraff
Copy editor Anne Newman
Editorial Assistant Cecilia Desmond
Production Geoff Barlow and Alice Holloway

A Cataloguing In Publication record for this title is available from the British Library.

Printed and bound by Martins the Printers Ltd, Berwick upon Tweed

To my wonderful mum –
in loving memory

Marilyn Glenville PhD is the UK's leading expert in nutritional health for women. She obtained her doctorate from Cambridge University and is a Fellow of the Royal Society of Medicine and a member of the Nutrition Society.

For over 25 years Dr Glenville has studied and practised nutrition, both in the UK and in the US. She has had several papers published in scientific journals, frequently advises health professionals and often lectures at academic conferences held at The Medical Society, the Royal College of Physicians and The Royal College of Surgeons. She is also a popular international speaker. As a respected author on women's health care she gives regular talks on radio and has often appeared on television and in the press.

Dr Glenville is the editorial representative on the Forum for Food and Health at the Royal Society of Medicine and is also on the Medical Advisory Panel for the registered charity, Women's Health. She is patron of the Daisy Network, a premature menopause support group. Dr Glenville was formerly an observer on the Foods Standards Agency's Expert Group on the safety of vitamins and minerals.

She is also the author of six internationally best-selling books on health including: *Natural Alternatives to Dieting*, *New Natural Alternatives to HRT*, *Healthy Eating for the Menopause*, *Natural Solutions to Infertility*, *The Nutritional Health Handbook for Women*, and *Natural Solutions to PMS*.

Dr Glenville runs her own clinics in London and Tunbridge Wells and also has a website: www.marilynglenville.com

Contents

Introduction

Can you answer 'yes' to any of these questions?

- Do you have a family history of osteoporosis?
- Are you of European or Asian descent?
- Have you ever yo-yo dieted or suffered from an eating disorder such as anorexia or bulimia?
- Were you prone to irregular menstrual cycles or long gaps between periods when younger?
- Are you (or have you ever been) a smoker?
- Have you taken certain medications – steroids, heparin, anticonvulsants, diuretics, long-term laxatives or antacids?
- Have you had a thyroid problem – either under- or overactive?
- Do you not take enough (or any) exercise?
- Do you exercise too much?
- Did you have an early menopause (before the age of 40)?
- Have you had a hysterectomy and had your ovaries removed?
- Do you have a digestive problem such as Crohn's, ulcerative colitis or coeliac disease?
- Is your alcohol and/or caffeine intake heavy (more than seven units per week or two cups of coffee or tea per day)?
- Are you underweight or slim and sma-boned?
- Have you already broken any bones?
- Have you become shorter with age?
- Have you never had children?
- Are you post-menopausal?
- **Are you a woman!?**

If so, you may be at risk of osteoporosis and this book is for you.

——————— **Note to reader** ———————

Strictly speaking, bone mass and bone density refer to different things. Bone mass is the total mass of the bone in the whole body (mass = density x volume); whereas bone density refers to the amount of bone in a particular area (e.g hip). However, the two terms are often used interchangeably in bone science literature, so for ease of reading, in this book, I have decided to use the term 'bone density'.

Similarly, the terms bone density and bone mineral density are interchangable, but I have chosen to use bone density.

Osteoporosis is a preventable illness affecting many more women than men – 1 in 3 women over the age of 50 in the UK and 1 in 9 men are sufferers. Public awareness and understanding of the illness, however, remains woefully limited: osteoporosis is not just a matter of brittle bones; it can kill – in fact it kills more women than ovarian, cervical and uterine cancers combined. Up to 20 per cent of women who suffer hip fractures die within six months of sustaining the fracture. Complications can arise from surgery, pain can be chronic and severe, and patients are hospitalised, losing their independence and often their will to live. Also, whilst osteoporosis is often thought of as an old person's disease, it can strike at any time. By about the age of 20 women have (or should have) acquired 98 per cent of their bone density; this then stabilises in their 30s and 40s, then it starts to fall. The decline is more rapid around the menopause and is faster in some women than it is in others. The severe pain, deformities and loss of independence that are consequences of bone loss are such that 80 per cent of women would rather die than suffer a hip fracture and be bedridden in a nursing home.

As well as the suffering it undoubtedly causes so many women, osteoporosis in the UK is also putting a major strain on the NHS, costing it £1.7 billion a year in diagnosis and treatment, a figure that is expected to rise to £2.1 billion by 2010. A national breast-screening programme offers a mammogram to every woman over the age of 50 every three years, and women are eligible for free mammograms until the age of 70. Yet despite the fact that osteoporosis is a major health problem affecting three times as many women as breast cancer, there is no osteoporosis-screening programme in place in the UK. Similarly, in the US where osteoporosis is considered a major public health threat for 55 per cent of people aged 50 years and older, less than one third of women defined as 'high risk' have their bone mineral density tested.[1]

Sometimes the first sign of osteoporosis is a fracture following a relatively minor bump or accident. It has even been thought that in many cases, the bone breaks first, causing the fall, rather than the other way around. For some women the first sign is a loss of height or kyphosis (one sign is an obvious dowager's hump) and some women do get symptoms of back pain, as the vertebrae in the spine start to collapse. However, one of the biggest problems associated with osteoporosis is that it is often also a 'silent disease', in which bone loss happens gradually over time, without any symptoms at all presenting. This is why early screening for osteoporosis could prove invaluable, given that it is essentially a preventable and treatable disease.

The World Health Organisation (WHO) has devised the following set of principles and practices[2] intended to serve as the basis for recommending or planning screening for early detection of any disease:

- The condition should be an important health problem.
- There should be an accepted treatment for patients with recognised disease.
- Facilities for diagnosis and treatment should be available.
- There should be a recognisable latent *(hidden)* or early symptomatic stage.
- There should be a suitable test or examination.
- The test should be acceptable to the population.
- The natural history of the condition, including development from latent to declared disease, should be adequately understood.
- There should be an agreed policy on whom to treat as patients.
- The cost of case-finding should be economically balanced in relation to possible expenditure as a whole.
- Case-finding should be a continuing process and not a 'once and for all' project.

> Out of every three women who suffer an osteoporotic fracture, only one recovers completely. Within one year of having a hip fracture, a third of women cannot live independently and 20 per cent die.

With these criteria in mind, I believe there is certainly adequate justification for a screening programme for osteoporosis.

In 2004, a leading medical journal ran an article entitled 'Osteoporosis screening – time to take responsibility', stating that the possibility of underlying bone loss must be addressed and that 'the status quo of "missed opportunities" is unacceptable'.[3] This is a good sign that at last the medical profession is sitting up and taking notice but it takes a long time for the medical profession to come round, as illustrated in the case of folic acid, which has taken more than 20 years to become a mainstream recommendation to prevent spina bifida in the baby for women who want to conceive.

But what lies behind this epidemic of osteoporosis? Is it a modern phenomenon that we can blame on our diet and lifestyles rather than on ageing and dwindling oestrogen levels after the menopause? Clearly something in our modern lifestyle is affecting the density and strength of our bones, and only now are we beginning to understand what that might be. The biggest concern is for the next generation of girls, of whom many will not even reach their peak bone density by the age of 25 because of lifestyle factors such as smoking, lack of exercise (being driven to school, sitting in front of the television and computers), poor diet (high intake of soft drinks, see chapter 5) and dieting due to media pressure to be stick thin.

Being informed about osteoporosis is even more crucial now that women have been told not to take hormone replacement therapy (HRT) on a long-term basis because the benefits to the bones do not outweigh the risks of breast cancer, heart disease and thrombosis, for example. The current recommendation is that women should take HRT for five years only to combat the short-term symptoms of the menopause, which does not address long-term issues such as osteoporosis.

All this does make for gloomy reading but it is important to remember, as stated earlier, that firstly, osteoporosis is preventable and secondly, if you already have it, it is treatable. But early detection is vital and until further action is taken by the powers that be, it really is down to you to take responsibility for your health and do whatever it takes to get screened for osteoporosis.

'Osteoporosis, once thought to be a natural part of ageing among women, is no longer considered age- or gender-dependent. It is largely preventable due to the remarkable progress in the scientific understanding of its causes, diagnosis and treatment. Optimisation of bone health is a process that must occur throughout the lifespan in both males and females. Factors that influence bone health at all ages are essential to prevent osteoporosis and its devastating consequences.'
The National Institutes of Health Consensus Development Conference Statement on Osteoporosis Prevention, Diagnosis and Therapy, March 2000

You may be reading this because you know that you have one or more of the risk factors for osteoporosis listed earlier. Or you may have been told that you have low bone density (osteopenia) and now want to know how to prevent this from becoming full-blown osteoporosis. Or you may already have had a diagnosis of osteoporosis and want to know what treatments are available and what changes you can make to your lifestyle in order to improve your bone health. All this and more is covered in the following chapters – it's just a question of awareness and action. Whatever you do, don't just sit there and wait for the first fracture.

Chapter 1

What is Osteoporosis?

The word osteoporosis literally means 'porous bones', that is bones filled with tiny pores, or holes. Your bones change constantly – being broken down and rebuilt as you go about your everyday life. In fact, your bone cells are so active that your entire skeleton is replaced approximately every 10 to 12 years. However, problems arise when the rate of renewal does not keep up with the rate of breakdown, the result being bone loss. When this continues over a period of years, osteoporosis occurs.

Knowing just how bone is built up and lost can make it easier to see what you yourself can do to keep your bones healthy and strong.

——— Good bone structure ———

Bone is made up of three different elements:

'*Cortical bone*': this is the dense outer layer, which the body renews and completely replaces every 10 to 12 years.

The '*trabecular*' layer: an inner, spongy layer with a faster turnover, being replaced every two to three years. There are large concentrations of trabecular bone in the wrists, ankles and hips, and these are the most common fracture sites. Although the spine also contains substantial amounts of trabecular bone, the vertebrae tend to be protected and strengthened by their unique shape.

Collagen: a framework of collagen (a major bone protein) gives bone flexibility and crystals of calcium and phosphorus which give the bone strength.

BONE METABOLISM

A number of different systems in the body are involved in the bone metabolism process.

- **Building bone** Bone is living tissue that is constantly being broken down and replaced. Old bone tends to be weak and renewal – known as 'remodelling' – is therefore vital for bone strength. Remodelling, involving two different kinds of cells and several hormones, is characterised by a process called 'coupling'. In this process old or damaged bone is slowly dissolved by cells called 'osteoclasts' and the cavity this creates is filled by new bone created by other cells called 'osteoblasts'. The formation is said to be 'coupled', because when old bone is removed, new bone is formed at exactly the same location.

- **Losing bone** The process by which the osteoclast cells dissolve old or damaged bone is called 'bone resorption' (they, literally re-absorb the bone). The cells are instructed by the parathyroid hormone, which is manufactured by the parathyroid glands, found in the neck. Simply put, the parathyroid hormone acts on the osteoclasts, which resorb bone.

  If our calcium intake drops (say, for instance, if we go for a while without consuming enough calcium in our diet) the parathyroid hormone detects the deficiency and tries to remove calcium from bone, circulating it around in the blood instead, to correct the imbalance. The hormone also acts to stop calcium being flushed out of your body via your urine and activates vitamin D so that you are able to absorb more calcium from your food. Parathyroid hormone activates vitamin D by acting on the kidneys to increase the conversion of vitamin D to its active form – calcitriol. But if you're not consuming calcium or vitamin-D-rich food your body is going to be fighting an uphill struggle, and you could be losing bone density.

- **Restoring bone** The osteoblast cells work hard at 'bone formation' – filling the cavities left by removal of the old bone. The hormone 'calcitonin', produced by the thyroid gland, also leaps into action, incorporating calcium into new bone.

——— Functions of the bone hormones ———

Calcitonin

Production is stimulated by high calcium and magnesium in the blood. It:
- inhibits osteoclasts (slowing down resorption)
- decreases blood calcium levels
- stops release of calcium from the bones.

Parathyroid

Production is stimulated by low calcium and magnesium in the blood. Oestrogen stops its production. It:
- acts on osteoclasts (dissolves old bone)
- increases blood calcium levels
- triggers the release of calcium from the bones.

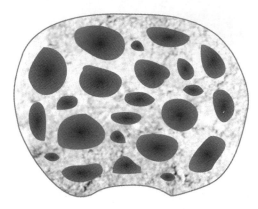

**Bone micro-structure
in a healthy bone**

**Bone micro-structure
in osteoporosis**

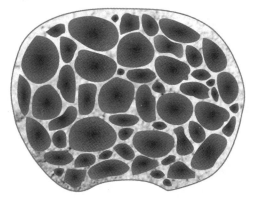

The bone renewal process also makes use of the sex hormones: a good supply of oestrogen helps both to stop the production of the parathyroid hormone which is removing calcium from the bones, and also to stimulate the release of the bone-building hormone, calcitonin. Testosterone too triggers the osteoblasts and increases levels of the enzyme that help to form calcium crystals in the bone.

Although oestrogen production in the ovaries slows dramatically at the menopause, sex hormones are also secreted by the adrenal glands which produce small, but extremely useful, amounts of oestrogen and testosterone plus a substance called 'androstenedione', which is converted to a form of oestrogen by body fat.

Finally, in addition to calcitonin, you also need both stomach (hydrochloric) acid (see page 107) and vitamin D in order to absorb calcium properly.

─────── **Bone remodelling through the years** ───────

Bone remodelling continues throughout your life but the balance between growth and loss changes with age. This is how it should look at different ages:

0–25: more bone formation than loss

25 (approx.): peak bone density – you have as much bone as you will ever have

30–40: the rate of bone formation is equal to the rate of loss – so your bone density is steady

40–50: steady but slow decline

Over 50: much sharper decline – bone loss is greater than bone formation so you start to lose bone density

PEAK BONE DENSITY

If your *peak bone density* is good at the age of 25 it makes sense that your bones will stand a better chance later on in life. Even though the menopause will trigger bone loss, you'll be in a strong position because you had more bone to begin with. So, the higher your *peak bone density*, the lower your risk of osteoporosis in later life.

Studies show that women who maintain good bone density right up to the age of 50 have a minimal risk of hip fracture later in life, compared with those who already have osteoporosis by the time they reach 50 and who have a 50 per cent risk of fracture as they get older.[1]

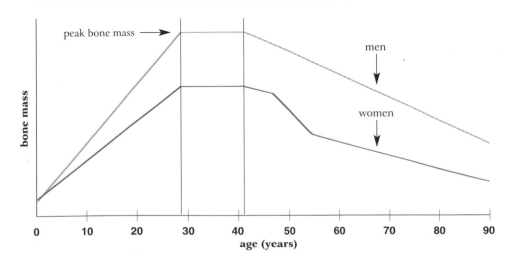

Genetic factors play a massive role in determining how good your peak bone density will be (accounting for as much as 50–80 per cent of the variation between different women) but the level is also affected by diet (how well you ate as a child), exercise, menstrual irregularities, chronic illness, and other factors such as eating disorders or taking steroids.[2]

Bone loss is, however, part of the normal ageing process but the problems arise when that bone loss is excessive. There are two different types of bone loss: that which occurs around the time of the menopause and is connected with increased osteoclast activity (more cavities are created making the bone more fragile), and the slower age-dependent bone loss which happens later in life to both men and women and is due to sluggish osteoblast activity, meaning that new bone is not formed.

Not every woman experiences a dramatic loss of bone after the menopause. A big trial investigating the impact of HRT on bone density found that 40 per cent of women who were not taking HRT had stable bones, yet some women who were taking HRT still lost bone.[3] However, some women can lose up to 20 per cent of their bone density in the five to seven years following the menopause, making them more susceptible to osteoporosis. The point is that we are all different, losing bone at different rates, which is why screening is so important.

Do women all around the world experience the same rate of osteoporosis?

The answer to this is definitely no, and one of the risk factors for osteoporosis is, in fact, ethnic origin (see chapter 2).

It has been found that there is a relatively low incidence of osteoporosis amongst African woman as compared with Asian and Caucasian women. African women seem to achieve a higher peak bone density in their early years before they start to lose bone.[4] Researchers have also found that Mayan women (in Mexico and Guatemala) live to a ripe old age of 80 without suffering from osteoporosis at all, and whilst there has been speculation that their oestrogen levels might be higher, this is not the case. In fact, in some cases they are lower than those in American white women. Bone density tests also show that that bone loss in Mayan women occurs at the same pace as it does in white American women. The only major difference is that their levels of testosterone (a hormone produced by the ovaries) remain constant before and after the menopause,[5] whereas in Western women these often drop post-menopause, potentially resulting in a reduced sex drive. In tests, it has been found that the male hormone testosterone triggers the bone-building osteoblasts, and this is accompanied by higher levels of the enzyme alkaline phosphatase, which helps to form calcium crystals in the bone. Certainly, men tend to experience far less bone-density loss than women.

IS OSTEOPOROSIS A NEW ILLNESS?

It has been suggested that women are not designed to live past the menopause and that nature intended us to expire at the demise of our fertile life. It is only because of the quality of life in the Western world, so this line of thinking goes, that we live on for another 30–50 years or more, and therefore carry a greater risk of osteoporosis.

This reasoning is supposedly supported by the fact that in other species of mammal the female dies at the end of her fertile years, obviously making the human menopause an aberration. But research shows that many mammals cease producing offspring well before the end of their life and in those that have been studied, it seems that although the females continued having cycles they did stop producing offspring in middle age, well before the end of their natural lifespan. So in fact women are not unique in enjoying a stage of life beyond their child-bearing years.

It is true that life expectancy was shorter centuries ago, especially for women. On the basis that 'average life expectancy' is calculated by adding up the ages at which people die and dividing that by the number of deaths, if many people die young, the average life expectancy will be low. In past centuries, many women died in childbirth, there was a high infant mortality rate and large numbers of people died through bad hygiene, poverty and malnutrition.

If you exclude these deaths (given that such causes are not prevalent today) records show that many women did, in fact, live long lives and without suffering from osteoporosis. The remains of a number of 18th-century Caucasian women discovered beneath a London church were examined, revealing not only that some had died in their 80s, but also that their bones were stronger and denser than those of both pre- and post-menopausal women today.[6]

We have to look at what is going on in our modern way of life that causes this major health problem. Women have always got older and oestrogen levels have always dwindled after the menopause, so we cannot simply say that this rise in osteoporosis is caused by these factors. We need to look seriously at our modern lifestyle, including factors such as diet, exercise, smoking and drinking.

Osteoporosis is a time bomb and something must be done about it now.

Chapter 2

Risk Factors

As you saw in the Introduction, several factors can increase your risk of developing osteoporosis. However, even if you find yourself saying yes to several questions on that list (I know I certainly can), osteoporosis need not be inevitable and whilst you may be unable to alter your history or your genetic make-up, there is plenty you can do to strengthen your bones through diet and lifestyle changes.

So let's now take a more detailed look at the risk factors for osteoporosis.

Your mother had osteoporosis

Your risk of osteoporosis is increased if your mother (or even your father) had it. It is possible, however, that their condition may never have been diagnosed in which case you need to look for clues: did they or other older relatives have a dowager's hump (an outward curving of the spine known medically as kyphosis) or did they lose height with age (due to the bones in the spine being compressed or crushed), for example? Think about whether there have been any changes to your own height too – are you finding that you have to stand on tiptoe to reach a cupboard that you could reach easily not so long ago?

The link between heredity and osteoporosis is being increasingly emphasised. By isolating the impact of heredity from that of lifestyle and environment on identical twins, research suggests that as much as 85 per cent of bone development may be genetically determined. Unlike non-identical twins, whose genes (and bones) are no more alike than those of ordinary siblings, identical twins of both sexes and all ages have almost matching bone density. The studies suggest that the genes that regulate bone influence both its peak density (the point at which bones are at their strongest) and the rate at which it is lost.

However, scientists believe that more than one gene may be involved and different 'candidate genes' are being investigated. The aim is to highlight those genes that control the way in which the body uses vitamin D (the vitamin D receptor or VDR gene), and to discover whether others can prevent the absorption of oestrogen (the oestrogen receptor gene), or if they are perhaps involved in the metabolism of collagen (a major bone protein).

The COL1A1 (Collagen type 1 alpha 1) gene has been identified as being the one that regulates collagen metabolism and a blood test has been devised to discover people who carry a mutation of the gene. The test can pick up this genetic marker in the blood and so predict fractures as effectively as bone scanning.[1] For more on the genetic aspects and screening of osteoporosis see chapter 8.

You are of European or Asian descent

Whilst osteoporosis is common amongst Asian and Caucasian women, African women are relatively immune. So, clearly, ethnicity is a factor. Furthermore, there are variations within racial groups showing that women from Northern Europe are more at risk than those from Mediterranean countries. But why is this?

An inactive lifestyle combined with a lack of sunlight, depressing vitamin D production, could explain the higher incidence of osteoporosis amongst the women of Northern Europe. Afro-Caribbean women, on the other hand, may have a natural protection. It is known that they are more susceptible to fibroids – benign growths in the womb that are known to be sensitive to higher levels of oestrogen. If Afro-Caribbean women are producing higher levels of oestrogen than Asian or Caucasian women, they may have an inbuilt resistance to osteoporosis.

You have or have had an eating disorder or disordered eating

Whilst the link between anorexia or bulimia and osteoporosis has been recognised for some time, scientists have only recently started to focus on a much more common phenomenon – women with disordered eating patterns. Dissatisfied with their bodies, and heavily influenced by relentless media exposure to emaciated models and celebrities, large numbers of women in the West routinely restrict their food intake in an attempt to control their weight. They do not have anorexia or bulimia, but their diet is affecting their health. One study showed that 37 per cent of Canadian women with a healthy body weight (BMI 20–24) were trying to lose weight.[2] Even amongst girls as young as 9 and 10, 40 per cent were dieting,[3] a trend continuing into their teens with a frightening 60 per cent restricting their food intake.[4]

Taken to its extreme, dieting can reduce body fat to the extent that periods stop. When this happens, bone health is undoubtedly affected. It was previously thought that in young women with anorexia nervosa the body did not have a chance to build up enough bone in the first place. However, more recent research suggests that bone formation is the same in anorexia sufferers as it is in healthy women of the same age, only they are losing bone at a much faster rate.[5] Researchers are not as yet entirely sure how anorexia affects bone density but they consider it to be a combination of factors including low weight, hormonal problems from irregularities in the menstrual cycle and malnutrition from restricted food intake. It is likely that there would be deficiencies of nutrients such as calcium, magnesium and zinc, which are essential for bone health. If you suffer (or have ever suffered) from an eating disorder or disordered eating you should ask for a bone density scan (see page 30) and do a bone turnover test (see page 32). Even if you have been healthy for a number of years your medical history may put you at risk of developing osteoporosis later on.

Your periods have been irregular

Women who experience irregular cycles or missed periods over several months lose a significant amount of the bone-protective effects of the normal circulating female hormones. A bone scan and bone turnover test (see pages 30 and 32) can help to find out exactly how things stand. Women with a history of irregular periods before the age of 40 have an average loss in bone density of more than 8 per cent compared to women with regular periods.[6]

You are (or were) a smoker

Smoking not only reduces bone density (by up to 25 per cent) but also increases the risk of hip fractures.[7] It can wreak havoc on the balance of female hormones by pushing a woman into an earlier menopause, so reducing her oestrogen levels.[8] Of women who have gone into the menopause before the age of 46, a large proportion are smokers.

You have taken certain drugs

Because some drugs can accelerate bone loss, you should ask your GP about the possible bone-related side effects of any medication you are taking (or have taken) long term. The following drugs can increase your risk of osteoporosis:

Steroid medication

Steroid medication has an effect on calcium absorption and decreases osteoblast (bone building) activity as well as causing more excretion of calcium, so these drugs have quite a dramatic effect overall on bone metabolism. They include:

• oral corticosteroids (such as prednisolone, if used for three months or more), prescribed for chronic inflammatory disorders such as rheumatoid arthritis or ulcerative colitis
• corticosteroids or glucocorticoids (such as cortisol, corticosterone, cortisone and hydrocortisone). They cause a reduction in bone formation

which can result in a 10 to 15 per cent overall bone loss and make fractures significantly more likely, both in the hip and spine. [9]

In December 2002 the Royal College of Physicians, in collaboration with the Bone and Tooth Society and the National Osteoporosis Society, published evidence-based guidelines on the prevention and treatment of glucocorticoid-induced osteoporosis.[10] The concern is that the risk of fracture is dependent on the dose of glucocorticoid, but an increased risk is being seen at doses of prednisolone less than 7.5mg per day. The risk of fracture is high soon after starting the steroids but goes down quickly after stopping treatment. If you are on or have had to take steroids in the past it is important to have a bone density scan and bone turnover test (see page 32).

There are also concerns that inhaled steroids, such as those taken by people with asthma, have a detrimental effect on the bones, showing that the more puffs per day a woman takes, the greater her bone loss.[11] Opinion seems to be divided as to whether inhaled steroids cause bone loss only in post-menopausal and not in pre-menopausal women,[12] so if you use or have used inhaled steroids and are over the age of 25, it is advisable that you have your bone density checked (see page 30). You should also make sure that you put into place all the diet and exercise recommendations in chapters 5 and 7.

Laxatives and diuretics

Regular use of these can increase your risk of osteoporosis because calcium and other essential minerals like magnesium are being excreted from the body.

Thyroid medication

Overactive thyroid (hyperthyroidism or thyrotoxicosis) is a condition characterised by high levels of thyroid hormone which increases bone turnover. The link between hyperthyroidism and osteoporosis is well known.[13] However, there could also be an increased risk of osteoporosis if you have been taking thyroid hormone for an underactive thyroid (hypothyroidism) at too high a dose for many years. It is important that you have your levels monitored to ensure you are taking the appropriate dose.

Heparin

This blood-thinning drug can also increase bone loss. It is increasingly used during IVF treatment and to help prevent miscarriage.

Anticonvulsants

These drugs, used to control epilepsy, can interfere with calcium and vitamin D metabolism. They cause an increased rate of bone turnover (see page 32), thus affecting bone density. It is recommended that anybody who is taking anticonvulsant medication should also be taking additional vitamin D.[14] Many doctors, however, are not aware of the association between anticonvulsant medication and bone disease and less than 10 per cent of neurologists recommend taking calcium and vitamin D to protect against the side effects of these drugs.[15]

Antacids

Used to control indigestion, reflux and dyspepsia, antacids – as the name suggests – work by decreasing stomach acid. However, good levels of stomach acid are, in fact, needed to absorb calcium (see page 107). Antacids also contain aluminium, which accelerates the excretion of calcium, and to compound the problem, some contain calcium carbonate – a form of calcium that is not easily absorbed and requires a good level of stomach acid for absorption. So, ironically, people take calcium-containing antacids often in the mistaken belief that they are benefiting from extra calcium, when in fact their stomach acid is lowered to the point where it can't adequately absorb it.

If you are taking antacids on a regular basis it would be advisable to have both a bone density scan and a bone turnover test to know where you stand at the moment and what action you need to take. Do not stop taking any medication without consulting your doctor. However, they may be able to suggest an alternative medication that does not have a negative effect on your bones. Some digestive problems can even be treated using nutritional medicine, i.e. a combination of diet and nutritional supplements.

You don't take much exercise

The more demand that is placed on bone the stronger it becomes. The work that your muscles do in everyday life stimulates your bones (at the points where the muscles connect to them) to strengthen themselves. And gravity itself puts your bones under pressure – astronauts lose bone density after a few months up in space without it. So bones that aren't stimulated into regular replacement are susceptible to osteoporosis. It's very much a case of use it or lose it.

The best form of bone-strengthening exercise is the weight-bearing kind which exerts pressure on the bones (see chapter 7). Whilst I would never advocate exercising to excess (see below), moderate exercise can help to increase bone density. Keeping yourself fit will also improve your co-ordination and flexibility, making you less likely to fall, and that, in turn, reduces the risk of fractures.

You exercise too much

Exercising to extremes can be as much of a problem as not exercising enough. Women involved in intense physical training, such as athletics or ballet dancing, often find that their periods stop because they have lost too much body fat and this puts them at risk of osteoporosis. Nature always favours a balance, so whilst it is essential to exercise, it is equally important not to overdo it.

You had an early menopause – medical or natural

Menopause normally occurs around the age of 50, but some women reach menopause at 40 or earlier.

Early menopause may sometimes be triggered by radiotherapy cancer treatment or by surgical removal of the ovaries (sometimes alongside a hysterectomy). If this is the case oestrogen levels will drop rapidly instead of declining gradually, as they normally would as you approach and enter menopause. Testosterone, produced by the ovaries, will also drop rapidly and this 'male' hormone plays an important role in bone metabolism as it triggers the osteoblasts (bone building cells) and increases levels of the enzyme that helps to form calcium crystals in the bone. This sudden drop in hormones can cause an alarmingly rapid rate of bone loss for more than five years afterwards.

Early menopause that is not brought on by surgery or radiotherapy affects an estimated 110,000 women in the UK, some still in their teens and early 20s. Periods can start normally and then suddenly stop. Premature menopause is usually diagnosed by a combination of blood tests and pelvic ultrasound scans. It can be devastating for a young woman to discover she has reached the menopause – not only does it render her infertile (unless she is able or willing to use donor eggs), it also means that she will have to cope with menopausal symptoms and possibly osteoporosis at a very young age. Until recently, this problem did not receive much attention; however there is now, fortunately, much greater awareness and an organisation called the Daisy Network (see page 182) has been set up to support women who are affected.

Any woman under the age of 40 who has experienced a surgical menopause (ovaries removed with or without a hysterectomy), had radiotherapy or discovered that she has gone through an early menopause naturally will need to discuss the use of hormone replacement therapy (HRT) with her doctor. Although I have been a vocal exponent of natural alternatives to HRT (see my book *New Natural Alternatives to HRT*), it is important to keep in mind that a premature menopause is a medical condition and one that could render a young woman short of the female hormones that are essential for her bones for up to 30 years longer than is normal.

If you have been through a premature menopause with no medical reason and a pelvic ultrasound scan shows that your ovaries look healthy, it is worth trying the natural approach to get your periods back. (This subject is covered in detail in my book *Nutritional Health Handbook for Women*.) The sooner you do something about the problem, the greater the chance that the natural approach will work – in other words, if you start treatment as soon as possible after your periods stop and your condition is diagnosed, it is more likely that your periods will return. Stress, whether physical (like extreme weight loss) or emotional (car accident, bereavement) can cause periods to stop so it is worth addressing the cause of the problem.

You have digestive problems

Your body will not absorb essential nutrients that keep your bones strong unless your digestive system is working efficiently and there are three main reasons why this might be the case:

Insufficient stomach (hydrochloric) acid

As we get older we all tend to produce less stomach acid and this can interfere with the effective absorption of calcium and other nutrients. It is estimated that about 40 per cent of post-menopausal women are severely deficient in stomach acid; so even if you are eating well and taking supplements, you could be fighting a losing battle if you are not properly digesting or absorbing them. Taking antacids is not a good idea as they frequently contain aluminium which binds to minerals including calcium, preventing them from being absorbed (see page 79). Instead, think about why you might be experiencing digestive problems in the first place. A simple stool test (which can be organised by post through my clinic, see page 183) can help to pinpoint the cause of your digestive problems.

Coeliac disease

An increasingly common digestive disorder, coeliac disease is caused by an intolerance to the gluten found in grains such as wheat, rye, barley and oats. Sufferers have white blood cells in their gut lining which are programmed to 'see' gluten as a foreign substance and so reject it.

Coeliac disease is characterised by weight loss and diarrhoea. This means that a number of essential nutrients simply don't get absorbed, thus increasing the risk of osteoporosis. Many sufferers are deficient in vitamins A, D, E, K, folic acid and other B vitamins, zinc and selenium. The disease also makes the absorption of calcium difficult, particularly if you are also deficient in vitamin D (see chapter 6).

Crohn's and ulcerative colitis

Both Crohn's and ulcerative colitis are classed as inflammatory bowel diseases where either the whole or parts of the intestines become inflamed. Symptoms can include diarrhoea, rectal bleeding and abdominal pain. Both Crohn's and ulcerative colitis can cause problems with the absorption of valuable nutrients from food and so can increase the risk of osteoporosis.

Your alcohol and caffeine intake is heavy

Both alcohol and caffeine can have a negative effect on bone health and this is covered in detail in chapter 11.

You are underweight or slim and small-boned

As you get older (particularly around the menopause), the ovaries slow their production of oestrogen. Your fat cells, on the other hand, continue to produce a weak form of oestrogen called oestrone which can help to protect against osteoporosis, but a certain amount of body fat is needed for adequate oestrone to be made. In today's society, women feel increasingly pressurised to be ultra-slim, but this clearly puts their bones at great risk.

When you are younger you also need a certain amount of fat in order to keep your periods going. Your body is very clever: when food is in short supply and your body believes it could be on the brink of death, it shuts down your reproductive system, being, as it is, the only system you don't need in order to stay alive. The body's resources are then channelled away from your reproductive organs and into areas in greater need. Your body also senses that there is not enough food to sustain both you and a baby, so it takes steps to prevent a pregnancy before it can happen – a sort of natural birth control. If your periods stop because you are underweight you won't have the protection of the circulating female hormones for your bones. This increases your risk of osteoporosis.

Unfortunately, being slim and small-boned, especially if you are Caucasian, is an automatic risk factor for osteoporosis, even if you have never dieted in your life. This is just a question of heredity and it means that you will need to do more to prevent osteoporosis than women with a larger build.

If you have a good appetite and are eating well, and yet you are underweight or have unexplained weight loss, you should consult your doctor – the weight loss could be due to a problem needing medical treatment. You may have an overactive thyroid and this can increase your risk of osteoporosis. If you have been checked medically and given the all-clear then it is worth looking for another approach. It may be possible that you are not absorbing nutrients properly or that you have an inherent problem such as a parasitic infection. Good digestion is crucial in the fight against osteoporosis because you need to be able to absorb adequate nutrients from your food and any supplements you are taking in order to feed your bones.

It is possible to perform a digestive analysis on a stool sample and find out how well you digest and absorb nutrients (this can be arranged through my clinic, see page 181). The test also evaluates whether you have hidden yeasts or bacterial or parasitic infections and whether you have enough beneficial bacteria.

You have already broken a bone

If you fell downstairs when you were younger and broke your leg, the fracture was obviously due to the high trauma of the fall and not the fact that your bones were osteoporotic. An osteoporotic fracture usually results from a low-trauma injury such as twisting your ankle. If you have already broken a bone in this way it may mean that you have osteoporosis but it has not been picked up or investigated thoroughly enough. With osteoporotic fractures, you have twice the risk of having another fracture if you have already broken a bone from a low-trauma injury and four times the risk of having another vertebral fracture if the first one was a vertebral fracture.[16]

That is why it is important to make sure that you see your doctor if you have experienced a low-trauma fracture so that a bone scan can be arranged and you can be monitored.

You are becoming shorter with age

If you have noticed that you are finding it hard to reach wall cupboards or other high places that you could reach before, then it is possible that you are losing height. This is important in relation to osteoporosis as it could indicate that the vertebrae in the spine are starting to collapse.

You have never had children

The general consensus from a number of studies is that women with a history of one or more children have a 2–5 per cent higher bone mineral density than those who have never had children.[17] It is thought that the months of high oestrogen levels during pregnancy contribute to higher bone density.

So if you have not had children and especially if you have any of the other risk factors listed, it is important to have a bone scan to find out where you stand.

You are post-menopausal

Bone loss begins around the age of 40, and dwindles at a rate of 0.5–1.0 per cent per year. As women enter the menopause, this rate increases to 2–5 per cent for the next 8–10 years. Some women, unfortunately, can lose up to 20 per cent of their bone density in the 5–7 years following the menopause, making them more susceptible to osteoporosis. We are all made differently. Even if you look and feel perfectly healthy, you could be losing bone at an alarming rate without knowing it. This is why testing is so important.

You are a woman

Just being a woman is a huge risk factor for osteoporosis. Seventy-five per cent of all hip fractures occur in women and 1 in 3 women will develop osteoporosis compared with just 1 in 9 men. Generally, women tend to be smaller boned and slimmer than men, and men produce testosterone all their lives (with no great middle-age drop), ensuring a continued triggering of the bone-building osteoblasts.

SO WHAT DO ALL THESE RISK FACTORS ACTUALLY MEAN?

Whilst certain factors or combinations of factors can increase your risk, it does not necessarily mean that you are going to get osteoporosis, it just increases the chances.

Information is invaluable because if you know that your mother had a hip fracture and you are in your early 40s but missed a year of periods when you were in your 20s, you have good indications that you should get a bone density scan and a bone turnover test now. You could adopt the ostrich technique and say that if your bone density is low, you'd rather not know about it. But remember that whilst osteoporosis is preventable, it is much harder to treat. Think of it in terms of a car MOT: your brakes are a bit low but getting them fixed now could prevent an accident later.

It is never too early to be screened for osteoporosis. Once you hit your 30s it is worth being checked out – if everything is fine, then you know that whatever you are doing is working and you just need to keep monitoring every two years; if the outlook is not so good, then by following the recommendations in this book you can work on prevention before osteoporosis takes hold.

Chapter 3

Testing for Osteoporosis

WHY TEST FOR OSTEOPOROSIS?

Looking at and identifying with the risk factors outlined in chapter 2 is one step towards being informed about osteoporosis and how it might affect you. However, this will not tell you whether or not you already have a problem. By having your bone health assessed, you will ascertain one of the following:

- your bones are normal and you need only work on osteoporosis prevention
- your bones are below normal (there is osteopenia but not osteoporosis), in which case the aim is to work on strengthening the bones in order to build up bone density and also to prevent the problem from getting worse and developing into full-blown osteoporosis
- you already have osteoporosis and need to consider the best possible treatment and lifestyle strategies.

Having as much information about your bones as possible will allow you to make informed choices as to the most appropriate approach for you, hopefully avoiding unnecessary drugs that may have uncomfortable side effects. And because bone density can be continually measured and monitored, you can form an ongoing assessment of your bone strength so that should the situation change you can adjust your plan accordingly.

What follows is a breakdown of the tests most commonly used to assess bone health.

DEXA scan

This form of scan is the most respected measure of bone density. Whereas an ordinary X-ray only shows osteoporosis where there is a 30–50 per cent bone-density loss (by which time it is almost too late) a DEXA (Dual Energy X-ray Absorptiometry) scan uses two X-ray energy beams. The low-energy beam passes through soft tissue but not bone, whilst the high-energy beam passes through both so that your bone density can be calculated by working out the difference between the two readings. The scanner measures bone density at many different points on the body. This is useful because a reading on part of the body does not necessarily reflect the situation at other points. With osteoporosis, bone loss typically starts in the trabecular bones (such as the spine and hip), so these are important sites to test first.

As with most things, there are some drawbacks to the DEXA scan. One is that it exposes you to X-rays, at the same intensity as a chest X-ray, and these are best avoided wherever possible. Also, the machine has to be operated by a radiologist and is only available in too few specialised units. Another disadvantage is that although both hip and spine are measured during a DEXA scan, conditions such as osteoarthritis and scoliosis, which is curvature of the spine, can give falsely high readings of bone density, making it difficult to estimate the spine's strength. (This can be a particular problem with the elderly or in people who have already sustained a fracture in the spine.) It is now accepted that the most accurate measurements are those from the hip.[1]

QCT scan

It is possible to measure bone density using quantitative computed tomography (QCT) scanners (also known as CAT scans). These give highly accurate measurements of bone density but at the same time they expose you to a high dose of radiation. They are also very expensive.

Ultrasound scan

The technology for using ultrasound to measure bone health has been developing rapidly over the last few years. In an ultrasound scan (also known as quantitative ultrasound scan or QUS scan), sound waves are passed through the heel (calcaneus) bone which, like the hip and spine, is rich in trabecular bone. QUS scans do not actually measure bone density (on which the WHO definition is based, see page 36) but measure other factors related to bone strength and quality such as stiffness and elasticity. However, recent research has shown that the QUS scans can predict those patients who will subsequently go on to have a fracture as well as DEXA scans,[2] and that they can 'predict early postmenopausal fractures as well or even better' than X-rays.[3] Furthermore, a recent study which looked at using QUS on younger women compared QUS with DEXA on women aged 20–39 years old and found that QUS worked as well as DEXA for identifying women at high risk of vertebral fractures.[4]

A number of QUS machines are available, some of which are more accurate and reliable than others. Whilst questions were raised concerning the accuracy and repeatability (i.e. that you can repeat the scan on the same day and get the same results) of first-generation QUS machines (because the technology performed a 'blind' measurement with no image to guide the practitioner), a new generation of QUS scanners now incorporates the same reference image that is normally seen in a DEXA scan. This image confirms that the person is positioned correctly.

QUS measurements are also temperature dependent, so some machines are susceptible to cold and can give variable readings. Thermally controlled water is the gold standard for ultrasound scans as they give consistency and precision.

I see ultrasound being used increasingly as a screening tool to help women of all ages to know whether they are at risk of osteoporosis. The scanners are easily portable, quick and convenient to use. They are safe, avoiding unnecessary exposure to X-rays, and relatively inexpensive compared to DEXA and QCT. The National Osteoporosis Society (NOS) is therefore suggesting that ultrasound be used as a screening tool to decide which women should go for a DEXA scan. This would mean that the DEXA is only used where absolutely necessary, eliminating avoidable risk and expense.

As with the DEXA scans, an ultrasound is normally repeated after two years (sometimes after one, depending on your situation).

Bone turnover blood and urine tests

Another way of assessing bone health is to measure microscopic biochemical markers (or 'clues') in blood or urine. Some of these show the rate at which bone is broken down (bone resorption) and others gauge the speed at which it is replaced (bone formation). Two of the markers that monitor the rate at which bone is broken down, N-telopeptide (NTx) and deoxypryridinoline, can be measured in a simple urine sample. At the moment NTx seems to be the more sensitive and specific, especially in women.[5] Higher levels of these bone resorption markers, indicating higher bone turnover and higher bone loss, have been found to be associated with a twofold increased risk of osteoporotic fracture.[6]

One of the markers for bone formation, alkaline phosphatase, is measured by a blood sample. Around the menopause, there is usually more bone being lost than built up, so the urine tests for bone resorption are more useful. And, as most osteoporosis drugs work by stopping bone loss, the urine tests can be used to monitor the effectiveness of the medication. This is the major advantage that bone turnover analysis has over scans (either DEXA or QUS): if you decide to take HRT or osteoporosis medication and/or start exercising and/or take supplements, this test can tell you whether your treatment is working. Bone turnover can be measured every three months and if what you are doing is effective, the bone turnover markers *will* go down. Where treatment or a new diet and exercise regime is not working, the test will again pick this up and another course of action can be suggested, whilst if it is working, it will give the necessary motivation to keep going. On the other hand, it can take a year, sometimes two, for a scan to register a lowering of bone density.

Bone turnover analysis is being used to predict the effectiveness of a group of osteoporosis drugs called bisphosphonates (see chapter 4). Changes in the 'clues' associated with bone turnover caused by the bisphosphonate drugs are not only linked with subsequent changes in bone density but can also predict the likelihood of future fractures. One study showed that patients treated with risedronate (a popular bisphosphonate) who showed a reduction in bone turnover markers at three months had a significant reduction in vertebral fracture risk. In fact, the analysis showed that the effects of risedronate on bone turnover were more important than the effects on bone density. The changes in bone turnover accounted for 66 per cent of the reduction in fracture risk whereas the changes in bone density only accounted for 26 per cent.[7]

The other benefit of bone turnover analysis is to monitor bone loss. In general, women lose about 1 per cent of spinal bone density per year during and after the menopause. But there is a group of women – around 35 per cent – who are known as 'rapid or fast losers' in that they can lose 3–5 per cent of bone per year. This loss could be picked up by bone turnover analysis because the markers would be fairly high.

Bone turnover analysis is important because bone density is not the be all and end all of bone health. Post-menopausal Chinese women, for example, have significantly lower hip bone mineral density than Caucasian women and are in theory at higher risk of osteoporosis.[8] Yet they sustain fewer fractures, probably because they have a lower rate of bone loss, which suggests that their rate of turnover is lower.

We do not routinely have bone scans at the age of 25–30 (when peak bone density is reached), so some women may have a constitutionally low bone density which has been low for years. If you were anorexic before the age of 25, or did very little exercise, or had to take steroid medication, for example, you may not have reached your peak bone density at the age of 25 and so your bone density in later life will be low. If your bone turnover is normal when tested it means you are not actively losing bone. This is important to know. It is far worse to have low bone density and a high bone turnover than to have a low bone density and a normal bone turnover.

There is no doubt that a measurement of bone turnover can give a useful perspective on the problem (see page 141 for more information on this test).

In my opinion, the bone turnover test is not used frequently enough in the diagnosis and treatment of osteoporosis. To get the full picture you need to look at your current rate of bone turnover together with your bone density. And, as stated above, it is also a crucial tool in monitoring the effectiveness of a given course of action so that you do not have to wait until the next bone density scan only to find that you have wasted up to two years on the wrong treatment plan.

Other tests

If you have been diagnosed with osteoporosis (especially if this has come out of the blue), and you don't really seem to have any of the risk factors listed on page 9, it would be worth asking for a referral to an endocrinologist (hormone specialist) as a number of endocrine glands can affect bone. A thorough screening by an endocrinologist can rule out any metabolic problems. Blood tests may include:

- serum calcium
- creatinine
- liver enzymes
- alkaline phosphatase
- thyroid profile
- osteocalcin levels
- hyperparathyroid assessment

───────── Limitations of bone density scans ─────────

Although bone scans can assess bone density, they cannot predict who is likely to sustain a fracture. Some women present with frighteningly low bone density – even into the osteoporotic range – and yet never suffer a fracture. Others record good bone density and still fracture.

An article in the *British Medical Journal* asked why doctors continue to measure bone density when analysis of 11 separate studies and over 2,000 fractures concluded that the scans 'cannot identify individuals who will have a fracture'.[9] The author argued that it might be more appropriate to measure bone turnover – the rate at which bone is lost – rather than bone density, because bone is a living dynamic tissue. 'Bone depends for strength more on its architecture than on its mass,' the article went on. 'If a bolt or two at a time were removed from a cantilever bridge for replacement, architectural strength might not be affected – but if a thousand were removed at one time (a high turnover state) architectural strength could be compromised critically, with little loss in mass.'

The glands that involve bone metabolism include the thyroid, parathyroid and pituitary.

Originally, the definition of osteoporosis was an actual fracture caused by having brittle, fragile bones. So in order to be diagnosed with osteoporosis, you would have already suffered a fracture. Now, as indicated by the definition on page 36, osteopororois is a label given to bone density that falls below a threshold arbitrarily defined by the World Health Organisation, and is essentially a risk factor for fractures. The WHO definition of osteoporosis is a warning that your bones may be more liable to break; it does not mean that they will. It would be the same as saying that you could predict that someone was going to have a heart attack because their cholesterol was high. High cholesterol is only one of many risk factors involved in heart disease – the information simply serves as a warning that you are at risk and therefore ought to take appropriate action. Also there are many people who have a heart attack and their cholesterol levels are within the normal range. This is the same dilemma we see with osteoporosis.

The dilemma of the predictive aspect of bone density scans was borne out by a study in 2004,[10] which asked how well do the World Health Organisation thresholds (that is the T score – see page 36) identify those women who will fracture. The study followed 149,524 for a year after having a bone mineral density scan. Eighty-two per cent of the women who had T scores better than -2.5 (i.e. they were not osteoporotic and seemingly had good bones) went on to have a fracture within that year. That is why I think it is so important that

---

CASE HISTORY

Sarah, aged 55, went to see her doctor complaining of slight pain in her back but only when bending forwards. Her diet was healthy, her weight was normal and she did not have any osteoporosis risk factors. Her menopause happened at the age of 51 and was very straightforward. Sarah's doctor suggested a bone density scan and the results showed a T score of -4.7 in her spine and -3.5 in her hip. A bone turnover urine test showed that she had a high rate of bone loss. So in the space of just a few weeks, Sarah went from thinking that she was relatively healthy to suddenly finding that her bone density was extremely low, she had a high fracture risk and she was still actively losing bone, for no apparent reason. Sarah was then referred by her doctor to an endocrinologist to have further tests, and at the same time she started a programme of supplements.

This illustrates just how important screening for osteoporosis is. Although Sarah was fortunate that the osteoporosis was picked up when she was still only 55, it would have been so much better had she had a routine ultrasound bone scan at the age of 40 so that action could have been taken to prevent the bone density from getting so low.

————————— **Measuring osteoporosis** —————————

To set the scene, the World Health Organisation (WHO) defines osteoporosis as a 'progressive systemic skeletal disease characterised by low bone mass and microarchitectural deterioration of bone tissue, with a consequent increase in bone fragility and susceptibility to fracture'.[11]

WHO then divides bone into three categories marked by 'standard deviations', units of variation used in statistics. The T score is the difference between your bone density and the average woman around the age of 25 at peak bone density (in other words how far off the ideal you are), whilst the Z score is your result compared with that of other women of the same age as you and is called 'age-matched' (that is, how you compare to your peers).

It is the T score that is used to determine whether you have osteoporosis:

Normal: T score = above -1.0 (that is -1.0 through zero to the plus numbers like +2.0 which are above average)
Osteopenia: T score = between -1.0 and -2.5
Osteoporosis: T score = less than -2.5

So if someone has a T score of -2 it means that they are twice as likely to have a fracture as someone with normal bone density. And within each grouping the lower the number the lower the bone density, so if two women have T scores of -3 and -4.5 respectively, it is the woman with -4.5 who has the more severe case of osteoporosis.

The T score of less than -2.5 applies to post-menopausal women and is a threshold at which treatment produces a reduction in the risk of fractures.[12] For pre-menopausal women and men the NOS has issued the following guidelines:

- If the T scores for the spine and total hip are both greater than -1.0 – then the results are normal.
- If at least one T score for the spine or total hip is less than -1.0 but both are greater than -2.5 then the scan shows osteopenia. Treatment may then be considered if:
- you have already had a low-trauma fracture or
- you are on steroid medication or
- you have a low (bone density) score for your age (Z score of less than -1.0).
- If at least one T score for spine or total hip is less than -2.5 – then the results show osteoporosis and treatment is recommended.

When retesting your bones, normally one or two years later, it is always better to repeat the scan on the same machine. The readings from bone density scans can vary as they are made by different manufacturers and may be calibrated slightly differently.

(**Note**: the WHO definitions of osteoporosis and osteopenia were originally developed for white females so this is not very helpful for women of other nationalities but the scores outlined above are now applied to all women.)

women also have a bone turnover test as well as a scan because these women who fractured without the diagnosis of osteoporosis could have had a high bone turnover, indicating that action should be taken immediately (to follow the lifestyle, diet and supplement recommendations in this book) in order to prevent that fracture in a year's time.

How to get your bones scanned

It's not easy to get a bone scan. Even if you have several of the risk factors listed on page 9, it can still be difficult to arrange. Chapter 9 – The Plan of Action for Osteoporosis – details what tests you need to do, including ultrasound bone scans and bone turnover and how you can get them done.

Chapter 4

Drug Treatments

In the bone metabolism process, as outlined in chapter 1, old bone dissolves to leave cavities which are then filled with new bone, creating a constant state of renewal which, in most young women, is perfectly balanced, so that no bone loss occurs.

Until recently, drug treatments for osteoporosis worked by preventing the loss of old bone; this does increase bone density and fractures are reduced, but the problem is that more old bone is kept in the skeleton, the quality of which is not as good as that of new bone. Now, however, there are two new drug treatments (teriparatide and strontium ranelate) on the market that can help to lay down new bone – this means better quality bone, because the improved bone density is coming from an increase in new bone rather than from preventing loss of old bone.

There are a number of drug treatments for osteoporosis, and they are as follows:

- Hormone Replacement Therapy (HRT)
- Selective Oestrogen Receptor Modulators (SERMs)
- Bisphosphonates
- Calcitonin
- Teriparatide
- Strontium ranelate
- Calcitriol
- Progesterone
- Statins
- Sodium fluoride

Let's now take a detailed look at all of these.

HORMONE REPLACEMENT THERAPY (HRT)

One of the main reasons why women have been persuaded to take HRT is for prevention of osteoporosis. However, it is important to realise that HRT carries risks, the biggest and most concerning of which is breast cancer. This is a classic situation in which it is extremely important to know the condition of your bones before embarking on a medication; if you have been told to take HRT for your bones you should ensure that you have a bone density scan and bone turnover test. If your tests are normal, then, in my opinion, it is not worth risking breast cancer in order to prevent osteoporosis, which can be avoided in most cases by benign measures such as diet and exercise. If your tests show osteoporosis, then you need to talk through with your doctor whether it is better to take a medication that is specifically designed for osteoporosis rather than HRT.

HRT has been around in different forms since the 1930s. Yet up until the Women's Health Initiative study in 2002 (see below) almost all the clinical trials focused on the impact of HRT on bone density without answering the question: does taking HRT reduce the risk of fractures?

The answer to this question is important. It is not enough to know that bone density has increased because we know that taking calcium along with vitamin D reduces the risk of fractures, but has little or no effect on bone density.[1] (And interestingly, there is a condition called osteopetrosis in which sufferers, who are born with the condition, have dense, but brittle bones which tend to fracture, indicating that good bone density does not necessarily mean fractures will be prevented.) That is why testing bone turnover is so important because it gives an indication of whether or not you are actively losing bone.

Only one randomised clinical trial before 2002 focused solely on HRT and fracture reduction[2] and in that one trial, the use of HRT did not show any statistically significant reduction in the number of broken bones.

The Women's Health Initiative study was the first large clinical trial to show that HRT did actually cause a significant overall reduction in osteoporotic fractures, with 35 per cent at the hip and 34 per cent in the spine.

So HRT does prevent fractures, but the effect is only temporary. When women stop taking HRT they tend to lose significant amounts of bone density. So if you go on HRT to prevent osteoporosis you would need to stay on it for ever and, of course, the risk of breast cancer from taking HRT increases the longer you stay on it.

One recent study compared the effects of stopping HRT with stopping one of the bisphosphonate osteoporosis drugs (alendronate, see page 43). The accelerated bone loss seen after discontinuing treatment with HRT was not evident after stopping alendronate. In fact bone density was maintained for one year after stopping alendronate.[3]

Another drug worth mentioning under HRT is tibolone (trade name Livial) – a no-bleed preparation available for post-menopausal women. It is a synthetic steroid compound that differs from the other HRTs in that it has some of the characteristics of oestrogen and progestogen but also has

————————— **HRT and breast cancer** —————————

The link between HRT and breast cancer has been known since 1976.[4] Numerous subsequent studies have confirmed this link and I have covered this aspect of HRT in detail in my book *New Natural Alternatives to HRT*.

In the summer of 2002 an eight-year Women's Health Initiative study in America was abandoned after five years because the benefits of HRT did not outweigh the risks. There was not only a higher risk of breast cancer from taking HRT but also a higher risk of heart disease and stroke.[5] The Million Women Study followed in August 2003,[6] the results of which were also damning. It suggested that use of HRT over ten years had resulted in an extra 20,000 cases of breast cancer, and that 15,000 of those were associated with combined HRT (oestrogen and progestogen). (This is the most common form of HRT used – only women who have had a hysterectomy use oestrogen without the progestogen.) The study has been criticised for overestimating the risk of breast cancer, but any way you look at it, the overall consensus from all the studies since the 1970s is that taking HRT carries an increased risk of breast cancer. The difficulty lies in measuring just how big that risk is.

androgenic or 'male' hormone qualities. It does not cause the changes in breast tissue that conventional HRT does, but because of its androgenic properties, it can cause an increase of facial hair as a side effect. It does seem to reduce bone loss but no study has, as yet, looked at whether it can reduce fractures, so taking it to prevent osteoporosis may not be wise.[7]

All the evidence indicates that if you have osteoporosis, there are more effective treatments than HRT (see chapter 6) and that for a woman who does not have osteoporosis 'the benefits of long-term treatment with oestrogen to prevent bone loss and fractures may not exceed the risk'.[8] It is interesting to note that in America, HRT is only approved by the FDA (Food and Drug Administration) for the prevention of osteoporosis, not for treatment of the disease.

————————— **Did you know...?** —————————

Since October 2003, HRT (Hormone Replacement Therapy) has been officially known as HT (hormone therapy). This is because scientists have recognised that these drugs are not 'replacing' the woman's own hormones and that the word 'replacement' implies risk-free, which is clearly not the case.

SELECTIVE OESTROGEN RECEPTOR MODULATORS (SERMS)

These are the new designer HRTs that are supposed to provide the beneficial effects of oestrogen where needed (in the bones, for example), whilst acting as an 'anti-oestrogen' in areas where too much oestrogen can be dangerous (such as the breasts and womb).

In our bodies we have receptors, which act as part of a lock and key system. Oestrogen travels in the bloodstream until it reaches the target tissue (for instance, the breasts). In order for the hormone to do its job, it has to be recognised by specific cells in the breasts called 'receptors'. Only those cells that possess 'oestrogen receptors' will respond to oestrogen. It's as if oestrogen is the key but it has to find the right lock in order to open the door.

There are two kinds of oestrogen receptors: alpha and beta. The alpha receptors are located in the womb, ovaries and breast. The beta receptors are found in the brain, blood vessels and bones, as well as the womb, ovaries and breasts.

Whilst conventional HRT seems to trigger the activity of both alpha and beta receptors all over the body, so causing stimulation of breast and womb tissue which could be triggering the increase risk of breast and womb cancer, SERMs block the alpha receptors in the breasts, womb and ovaries (thereby stopping excess stimulation of the cells in those areas) but have a positive, stimulating effect on the beta receptors in the bones, brain and blood vessels.

Raloxifene

One of the newest SERMs is raloxifene, used for the prevention and treatment of osteoporosis. Like conventional HRT, raloxifene has been shown to increase bone mineral density in women after the menopause.[9] It also reduces the risk of spinal fractures in post-menopausal women who already have osteoporosis,[10] but does not reduce the risk of fractures in other areas, such as the hip.

Further research has looked at whether raloxifene is helpful for women who only have osteopenia (low bone density) as opposed to those who have a diagnosis of osteoporosis. It seems that raloxifene significantly reduces the risk of vertebral fracture independent of the woman's starting level of bone density.[11]

Side effects

Many women, worried about the risks of taking conventional HRT, have been turning to raloxifene as a preventative drug for osteoporosis. But with this increased use it is important for women to know how well the drug is tolerated. One possible side effect is an increased risk of clots and so the drug is contraindicated for women at risk of deep vein thrombosis.

A study in 2004 in the medical journal *Osteoporosis International* looked at information collected from 13,987 women who had been prescribed raloxifene by their GPs and had been taking it for six months.[12] Flushing, one of the known side effects of raloxifene, was the most reported symptom and often the reason given for stopping taking it. Other symptoms mentioned as the women started the treatment included headache/migraine, nausea/vomiting, sweating, cramps, abdominal pain, dizziness, mastalgia (breast pain) and vaginal haemorrhage. There were 13 reports of deep vein thrombosis, 13 of a pulmonary embolism, 31 of thrombophlebitis (inflammation of a vein) and 29 of visual disturbances.

Notwithstanding these side effects, the report concluded that raloxifene is generally well tolerated. Should you experience any of them, however, you should think carefully about whether or not to continue taking it and perhaps seek your doctor's advice in this regard.

BISPHOSPHONATES

Bisphosphonates were originally used in industry as water softeners and anti-scaling agents, since they prevented the formation of calcium carbonate crystals. Now they are widely used as non-hormonal 'anti-resorptive' drugs, in the treatment of osteoporosis.

The bisphosphonates in use are:

- Etidronate (also known as Didronel)
- Alendronate (also known as Fosamax)
- Risedronate (also known as Actonel)

They work by inhibiting osteoclast (bone-dissolving cells) activity, which means that they stop the loss of old bone. The drugs are absorbed by the osteoclasts, inhibiting their activity and so reducing bone turnover. They can also stop osteoblasts (bone-building cells) from working, which is not ideal, but because they slow the loss of old bone, the bones remain in the same state for longer, so the drugs have the net effect of increasing bone density. Bisphosphonates actually get bound into one of the most important building blocks of bone (the hydroxyapatite crystals) within the bone matrix and so effectively alter the mineralisation process.

At the moment nobody knows what the optimum length of treatment should be for bisphosphonates. Nor is known the exact point at which their effects on the bones change from positive to negative. It has been suggested that bisphosphonates should only be taken for four to five years as they never leave the body after that period anyway. The 'half life' in bone is thought to be greater than ten years; this means that in ten years, about half of the amount of drug taken over that time will still be in the skeleton.

In view of this, if you have osteoporosis and require medication, I would suggest that the new drug, strontium ranelate (see page 46), would be a better choice.

Etidronate

This drug has been available for more than 30 years. To take it you need to follow a strict regime as you cannot eat for two hours before and after swallowing the tablets. This is because the drug is poorly absorbed and any food or other vitamins and minerals taken at the same time can prevent it from working. Also, etidronate is taken in cycles of 14 days followed by 76 days on a calcium supplement because etidronate tends to bind to bone. Taking it continuously and in high doses as it was prescribed 20 years ago can result in soft bones (osteomalacia).

Etidronate has not been approved in the USA as a treatment for osteoporosis but is widely used today in Europe and in Canada.

Research shows that etidronate increases bone density in both the hip and spine and that it does help to reduce vertebral fractures.[13] There is no information available as to whether or not it helps to reduce hip fractures.

Side effects

Side effects of this medication can include nausea, diarrhoea, skin reactions, headaches and constipation.

Alendronate

Alendronate is 700 times stronger than etidronate,[14] and can reduce the risk of fractures in both the hip and the spine in post-menopausal women with osteoporosis.[15]

A study called the Fracture Intervention Trial[16] compared the effects of taking daily alendronate on women who had already had a vertebral fracture and women whose hip bone-mineral density measurements were in the osteoporosis range but who had not had a fracture. After three to four years, alendronate reduced the risk of vertebral fractures by about 45 per cent for all the women in the trial regardless of whether they had already experienced a vertebral fracture.

Since 2001, alendronate has been available as a treatment for osteoporosis that is taken just once a week.

Side effects

The down side of taking alendronate is that it can cause digestive disturbances. It has to be taken on an empty stomach followed by at least 30 minutes remaining upright because it can irritate the oesophagus (the tube leading to the stomach). There have also been some reports of musculoskeletal aches and pains.

Risedronate

Risedronate is 1,000 times stronger than etridronate. It has been shown to increase bone density and to reduce most fractures by 39 per cent over three years.[17] It is used in women who are at high risk of osteoporosis and helps to reduce the likelihood of spinal damage in post-menopausal women who have already had a fracture.

Like alendronate, risedronate is also available as a medication that can be taken just once a week.

Side effects

The side effects from risedronate are also predominately digestive and can include inflammation and ulceration of the oesophagus. As with alendronate, special instructions about remaining upright and taking it on an empty stomach are given in order to try to reduce the side effects. Joint pains, nausea and stomach pain are other reported side effects.

Bisphosphonates, calcium and vitamin D

All the approved bisphosphonate treatments for osteoporosis have been tested alongside calcium and in most studies with vitamin D, so any increase in bone

---

—————— Weighing up bisphosphonates ——————

As seen above, bisphosphonates work by stopping the loss of old bone, and over time the mineral content of the bone increases. But scientists are beginning to wonder whether this increase in mineralisation is such a good thing.[18] Of course, the higher the mineral content, the stiffer the bone which means, in theory, it can withstand more stress. But if it becomes too highly mineralised, the bone can become brittle and cracks develop.

Regarding one of the bisphosphonates, some scientists have voiced the following concerns: 'There is no doubt that alendronate increases bone strength and decreases fracture rate during the first four years of use, but after that, the profound suppression of the bone formation rate may begin to have a negative effect'[19]. One study showed that women taking the drug for seven years had three times more spinal fractures than during the first three years even though their bone density had increased.[20] Another study showed that taking alendronate for ten years did not increase the fracture risk. However, the findings from this study were based on an estimate of fractures in the placebo group rather than actual fractures, so a true comparison of whether alendronate increased fractures is not possible from this study.[21]

density and reduction in fracture was always seen in the presence of adequate calcium and vitamin D.[22] If you are taking bisphosphonate treatment, therefore, it is important that you also take a supplement containing both calcium and vitamin D for maximum benefit.

CALCITONIN

Calcitonin, a natural hormone produced by the thyroid gland, inhibits the cells that break down bone (osteoclasts) and so makes the osteoblasts (bone-building cells) more effective. It is also found in some fish (e.g. salmon), as it helps to regulate their adaptation from seawater to fresh water.

Studies show that calcitonin does increase bone density and decreases the risk of fracture in both the hip and spine but not as effectively as the bisphosphonates.[23]

It used to be available in injection form but can now be obtained as a nasal spray.

Side effects

The main side effect seems to be nasal irritation and runny nose (rhinitis).

TERIPARATIDE

In 2002, the FDA in America approved a new drug for osteoporosis called Forsteo (called Forteo in the USA; generic name teriparatide) and it is now available in the UK. It is based on part of the parathyroid hormone which is responsible for both building and breaking down bone; scientists have isolated the bone-building element and developed it, so that the drug activates bone building in women who are taking the drug.

Until the introduction of teriparatide, none of the osteoporosis drugs actually helped to build up new bone (bisphosphonates are anti-resorptive drugs which only reduce the rate at which old bone is broken down). Because teriparatide stops osteoporosis by allowing new bone to grow at a faster rate, the quality of bone is better. Theoretically, the drug actually reverses osteoporosis.

Teriparatide is administered by self-injection once a day, into the skin of the thigh or abdomen and has been shown to reduce significantly fractures in both the spine and hip when taken along with calcium and vitamin D supplements.[24] However, because the long-term effects of this drug are not yet known, it should not be taken for more than two years. It is also very expensive at more than £5,000 for 18 months treatment in the UK and $500 for a 30-day supply in the USA.

Side effects

As with any drug, there are always side effects and the risks versus the benefits have to be weighed up. With teriparatide, studies on animals have shown that it increases the risk of osteosarcoma (bone cancer) although no incidence has been reported in human studies. However, the FDA state that 'the possibility that humans treated with teriparatide may face an increased risk of developing this cancer cannot be ruled out.'[25] Other reported side effects can include nausea, dizziness and leg cramps.

STRONTIUM RANELATE

This new treatment for osteoporosis is based on the chemical strontium, found in soil and water. Strontium ranelate (trade name Protelos) is the only drug available as yet which combines the slowing down of bone loss together with the building of new bone. Strontium ranelate is the first of a new class of drugs called DABAs (Dual-action Bone Agents). The advantage of the dual-action effect is that the drug should promote healthy new bone rather than just holding on to old bone as with the bisphosphonates, so the quality of bone should be better.

Studies have shown that strontium ranelate reduces the risk of spinal fracture by half after one year and by 41 per cent after three years,[26] as well as reducing the risk of hip fracture by a third over three years.[27]

Protelos is taken as a powder dissolved in cold water, best taken at bedtime at least two hours after eating to increase absorption.

Side effects

The most common side effects are diarrhoea, nausea, headaches and skin irritation. There does not seem to be the same degree of digestive problems that are often seen with the bisphosphonates. One other possible side effect is a blood clot, so if you are prone to clots it would be better to use another medication

CALCITRIOL

This drug is a synthetic version of the naturally occurring calcitriol which improves calcium absorption from the gut and aids the metabolism of calcium into bone. Calcitriol is an active form of vitamin D and vitamin D is essential for calcium to be absorbed by your bones.

Unfortunately, with this drug, which is taken in capsule form, the research does not agree as to whether it actually helps bone loss and reduces fractures.

Side effects

Side effects can include nausea and diarrhoea.

PROGESTERONE

Progesterone is a hormone naturally produced by the ovaries. It is the most important female hormone in the second half of the menstrual cycle and is absolutely necessary to maintain a pregnancy – a woman who is not producing sufficient progesterone when the egg is fertilised could miscarry.

Progestogen (or progestin, as it is known in the USA) is a synthetic form of progesterone, used in both the Pill and combined HRT, where it prevents the womb lining from building up excessively.

As they approach the menopause, many women will have periods without ovulating. Where ovulation is absent, progesterone is not produced in that cycle, leaving a dominance of oestrogen. Added to this, industry today constantly bombards us with xenoestrogens – foreign oestrogens – derived from petrochemicals and found in packaging, plastics and foods. An increasing number of disturbing developments are blamed on these chemicals and they are believed to have a devastating effecting on fertility, reproduction and health in both humans and animals. Studies have also linked xenoestrogens to the increase in breast and testicular cancers and to other oestrogen-dependent conditions such as endometriosis and fibroids.

The thinking behind the use of progesterone is that it should counterbalance the excess of oestrogen resulting from all of the above.

The first study to put progesterone into the bone health spotlight was conducted in 1990 by Dr John Lee, one of the foremost advocates of progesterone.[28] Women rubbed in progesterone cream to the softer skin under the arms, neck and face and the conclusion was that progesterone reduced the risk of fractures and increased bone density. But in this study, the hundred women being tested used progesterone in an 'Osteoporosis Treatment Programme' recommended by Dr Lee which also included:

Vitamin D	350–400ius per day
Vitamin C	2,000mg per day in divided doses
Beta-carotene	15mg per day
Calcium	800–1,000mg per day through diet and/or supplements
Oestrogen	0.3-0.625mg per day, 2 weeks per month (unless contraindicated)
Progesterone	3 per cent cream, applied twice daily, the last 12 days of the monthly cycle

The women were also told to: emphasise leafy green vegetables in their diet; limit red meat; restrict soft drinks (to three or fewer per week) and alcohol (none, or no more than one drink every two weeks); exercise for 20 minutes daily, or half an hour three times per week; not smoke any cigarettes.

Even though the women taking part in the study were making considerable changes in their regime, as outlined above, Dr Lee nevertheless concluded that it was the progesterone that was responsible for the difference in their bone. I would suggest that the improvement could well have been caused by the other factors. Notwithstanding this, many women have been treating themselves as guinea pigs and using progesterone for their bones since this study.[29]

One reason why women choose to use progesterone rather than any other drug is because they assume it is a natural product. However, this so-called 'natural' progesterone is synthesised (basically, man-made) from wild yam (a herb) in the laboratory. It can also be synthesised from soya. The word 'natural' in front of any product can be very misleading. Synthesising, or creating something that is chemically identical, does not make it 'natural'. In this context, it simply refers to a product that is identical to the hormone that your body produces from your ovaries, but is not natural in the real sense of the word. Don't be fooled. You could not eat wild yam or put it on your skin and expect your body to change it into progesterone.

If you choose a natural progesterone product (for example, a cream), make sure you are clear about the facts. You are taking a pharmaceutical hormone which constitutes HRT (hormone replacement therapy), only in this case it is progesterone, as opposed to oestrogen that you are replacing. A whole chapter is devoted to progesterone in my book *New Natural Alternatives to HRT*, simply because of confusion over this issue of 'natural' progesterone.

STATINS

This might seem a strange drug to include in a book on osteoporosis. Statins are a class of drugs used to lower cholesterol. They work by acting on an enzyme in the liver that controls the production of cholesterol. Only 50 per cent of cholesterol comes from your diet, the rest is produced by your liver.

Scientists have observed that older women taking statins to lower cholesterol had lower risks for hip and non-spine fractures. But the research to date which has actually asked the questions, do statins increase bone density and do they prevent fractures, is very confusing. One study in 2004 looked at whether statins were associated with higher bone density[30] and concluded that they were. However, this study was conducted through telephone calls to women who had come in for bone density scans, asking them what medication they were taking. A cause and effect relationship with the statins cannot be proven on this basis.

In another study in 2004, which was a double-blind randomised control trial, scientists found that the statin caused no changes in bone density in the spine or hip and the only increase was in the forearm. They concluded that the results did not support a general beneficial effect of statins on bone.[31] And as to whether statins prevent fractures, the answer seems to be no, judging by the results of a large analysis in 2004 of four prospective studies together with a meta-analysis of eight observational studies and two clinical trials that reported statin use and fracture outcome.[32]

Taking statins for osteoporosis is a big leap, especially as there is no evidence it will help your bones. And for high cholesterol my recommended approach would be to use nutrition and supplements because the statins do not address the problem of why your cholesterol is high in the first place. As soon as you stop taking them the problem recurs. The ultimate aim, surely, should be to get your body to stop producing the extra cholesterol in the first place and to lower the intake from your diet.

Some researchers are suggesting that the benefits of statins on heart disease are not only because they lower cholesterol but also because they have an anti-inflammatory effect;[33] this is very interesting given that other research shows that increased inflammation in the body leads to increased bone breakdown[34] (see chapter 8).

For women, there is another concern with statins. A large trial looking at the effects of statins on cholesterol found that there were 12 cases of breast cancer in

---

——————— Statins and co-enzyme Q10 ———————

If you are taking statins you should be aware that whilst they block the liver's ability to produce cholesterol, they also block production of co-enzyme Q10, an important substance found in all the body's tissues and organs. It is vital for energy production and helps to keep the metabolic processes working efficiently. It has also been suggested that it may have a role in preventing cancer and heart disease, lowering blood pressure and slowing down the ageing process. Unfortunately, however, co-enzyme Q10 declines with age and just 14 days on a statin can cause a further marked decrease in blood co-enzyme Q10 levels.[35]

Co-enzyme Q10 is crucial for healthy heart function. In one study, 84 per cent of patients with heart failure showed significant improvement when 100mg per day of co-enzyme Q10 was included in their treatment.[36] Q10 has also been given to patients waiting for a heart transplant where the waiting list is long and the number of donors small. These patients, with end-stage heart failure, were given 60mg of co-enzyme Q10 a day which resulted in significant improvements in the patients' symptoms, functional status and quality of life.[37]

To conclude, anyone on statins should be taking 50–100mg co-enzyme Q10 every day.

the women taking statins compared with only one case in the placebo group.[38] It was suggested that this could be due to chance and recent research is showing that those using statins have a lower risk of developing cancer.[39] However, this recent research was not a double-blind placebo-controlled trial but a study looking at the incidence of cancer in those already taking statins.

Side effects

Statins are powerful drugs and as with any medication have possible side effects which can include nausea, diarrhoea, constipation and muscle aches. (The blocking effect on co-enzyme Q10 – see page 49 – could explain the muscle aches and other muscular problems.[40]) Occasionally statins can cause problems with the levels of liver enzymes so these should be monitored.

SODIUM FLUORIDE

Fluoride was first used as a treatment for osteoporosis in 1966. It is an approved osteoporosis treatment in several countries, including France and Germany (although not in the UK or the USA as there is no evidence to show it reduces the risk of fractures). Until the development of teriparatide (see page 45) this was the only medication to stimulate bone formation directly as all other treatments were antiresorptive, meaning they just prevented bone loss. However, although studies suggest that fluoride triggers large increases in bone density, nobody knows whether this new bone is as strong as it should be and current evidence suggests that it does not lead to a subsequent reduction in fractures. As the Department of Health's Committee on the Medical Aspects of Food (COMA) has pointed out, the incorporation of fluoride into bone disturbs the alignment of the crystals, making the bone structurally weak and even more fragile than the existing bones.

What about fluoride in water? In the UK, most of the water is not artificially fluoridated and where it is, the rate is 1.5 parts per million (ppm) compared with 2 parts per million in the USA. When it occurs naturally, fluoride is derived from the minerals the water passes through and occurs at levels of around 0.1–2 ppm. High levels can increase the risk of hip fractures.[41]

The highest dose of fluoride you are likely to encounter is in toothpaste, where it can reach extremely high levels of 1,000 ppm. Excess fluoride cannot cause tooth loss because, unlike bone, enamel and dentine are not constantly being broken down and built up again, but it can lead to dental fluorosis, where the teeth are visibly pitted and stained. (Of course, there could be problems if swallowed in excess amounts.)

Side effects

Treatment with sodium fluoride can cause gastric irritation, vomiting and pains in the legs.

DRUGS IN THE PIPELINE

In the next five years, there will be more choices in terms of drugs for treating osteoporosis. Two new bisphosphonates are being developed, ibandronate (trade name Bonviva – which will be taken just once a month) and zoledronate (trade name Zometa). Although these will not differ markedly from the bisphosphonates already available, the aim is to give more choice in the ways and frequency with which the drugs can be taken, i.e. injection rather than tablet and the possibility of taking them monthly, quarterly or even yearly.

Two new SERMs are being developed – lasofoxifene and bazedoxifene – to help with menopausal symptoms and to treat breast cancer, with the bonus that they also have an impact on osteoporosis.

A skin patch is also being developed using the same substance as the medication Forsteo, but which would allow the drug to seep in through the bloodstream rather than being injected.

CHOOSING YOUR TREATMENT

The following table should help to make it easier to weigh up the information you have read in this chapter. It shows whether the drug can prevent fractures and in what parts of the body. A ✓ shows that the evidence is good, a + that the evidence is there, but not as strong as the ✓, and NS (not shown) indicates that the drug has not been shown to be effective.

Drug	Spine	Hip	Other non-vertebral fracture (e.g. wrist)
HRT	✓	+	✓
Tibolone	NS	NS	NS
Raloxifene	✓	NS	NS
Bisphosphonates	✓	✓	✓
Calcitonin	✓	+	+
Calcitriol	✓	+	+
Teriparatide	✓	✓	✓
Strontium ranelate	✓	✓	✓

What if you are a pre-menopausal woman with osteoporosis?

All the research so far has been focused on menopausal women (to whom the above table applies). But if you had anorexia as a teenager, or have been taking oral steroids for asthma for years, a bone density scan in your 30s could reveal osteoporosis. Are the above osteoporosis drugs effective for you and – more importantly – should you take them?

—— **Making informed decisions about drug treatments** ——

As with any treatment, the benefits need to outweigh the risks, and this is important when you are deciding on the best treatment for osteoporosis. Here are some tips:

- Find out whether a drug that has been prescribed is licensed for the *treatment* of osteoporosis or merely for the *prevention* of the disease. If you've already been diagnosed with osteoporosis there is no point in taking a drug that is not licensed for and more importantly does not treat osteoporosis.
- Some drugs only prevent fractures in one part of the body (such as the spine). Does the drug you are considering work on preventing hip, spine and other fractures such as the wrist, or is it really only beneficial for certain types of fractures? If you only have osteoporosis in the hip you may be wasting your time taking a drug that only works on the spine.
- Check that you are looking at treatments appropriate for your age group. If you have pre-menopausal osteoporosis you need to establish whether or not the drug prescribed for you has actually been tested on pre-menopausal women, as some are only tested on those who are post-menopause.
- Is there strong enough evidence to show a drug's effectiveness against osteoporosis to outweigh the risks of taking it? Consider the case of HRT, for example (see page 38).

At the moment there is no overall agreed treatment for young women with osteoporosis. What we do know is that if you are pre-menopausal and have osteoporosis as a result of taking steroids then the bisphosphonates can prevent bone loss. It is not known whether young women with osteoporosis from other causes will benefit from taking bisphosphonates. The other dilemma is that these drugs can stay in the body for up to ten years so they should be used with caution in young women.[42] Bisphosphonates may cross the placenta and the concern is that they could cause abnormalities in the skeleton of a baby should the woman become pregnant.

If you have gone through a premature menopause either because of surgery where the ovaries have been removed, or you have experienced what is called premature ovarian failure where your periods just stopped, you should speak to your doctor about HRT. Because menopause happens so early, a young woman would be short of essential female hormones for up to 30 years longer than is normal. These hormones are important for the bones as well as for preventing many of the other symptoms that can occur around the menopause, such as vaginal dryness and hot flushes.

Early HRT should not put young women at greater risk of breast cancer (see page 38) – experts believe it is the lifetime exposure to oestrogen that is significant. So women who start HRT in their late 30s or 40s due to an early menopause are not increasing their length of exposure to the hormone because they are only replacing the oestrogen that would have been manufactured and circulated by their body if they had not gone through the menopause. Young women with a premature menopause are really taking hormone *replacement* therapy: they are replacing the hormone that should have been there but is not. It is women who are going through the menopause at the usual age (average in the UK is 51) who should not be 'replacing' any hormones, because they are at a stage in their lives when the body is seeking naturally to reduce them.

It is thought that all the risks associated with HRT such as breast cancer, coronary heart disease, stroke, deep vein thrombosis, cancer of the womb lining and possibly ovarian cancer are connected with taking it after the menopause. The major problem with HRT in this context, however, is that at the moment there are no research studies to show whether it is effective for bone protection after early menopause.[43]

If you are young and have been given a diagnosis of osteoporosis, it is doubtful whether an osteoporotic drug treatment is appropriate. For you, the risk of breaking a bone is low and as bisphosphonates cannot be taken indefinitely, to take them now would limit your choices of drug treatment later and make the risks greater. Instead, you should focus on all the nutritional and exercise recommendations in this book and have your bones regularly monitored.

The situation is different, however, if you are young and have already suffered a low-trauma fracture (that is, one in which the broken bone does not seem justified by the fall – rolling over on your foot and breaking your ankle is not justified and would be classed as a low-trauma fracture). In this situation bisphosphonates could be useful in preventing another fracture – but you would need to avoid pregnancy while you are taking them.

No one knows whether other drugs like calcitriol and calcitonin are helpful for young women with osteoporosis, and other drugs like teriparatide are too new to be appropriately proven.

IN CONCLUSION

The emphasis with osteoporosis should, ideally, be on prevention, and this can be achieved using a combination of diet and exercise, as outlined in the chapters that follow. If you already have osteoporosis then the best medication around at the moment seems to be strontium ranelate. It carries few side effects and also seems to be producing better-quality bone – which makes it one up on the drugs that merely stop bone loss.

And no matter what medication you are given if you have osteoporosis, all the dietary recommendations and exercise should still be put into place because these can make the drug treatment more effective.

—— National Institute for Clinical Excellence (NICE) ——

NICE is a government body in England set up to provide advice to doctors on the effectiveness of certain drugs for particular medical conditions. As well as the effectiveness of the drugs, NICE has to decide whether a particular treatment is cost effective, in that the benefits of the drug outweigh the financial cost.

At the end of 2003, draft guidance was issued concerning the treatment of osteoporosis. This caused major concern as the recommendation was that there would be no drug treatments for post-menopausal women with osteoporosis and at high risk of fracture unless they have already suffered a fracture. In effect, this restriction would mean that nobody would be treated for prevention. The other proposals were that women over the age of 65 should be treated with osteoporosis drugs if they had a 'fragility fracture' but without having a bone scan first. Experts did point out that osteoporosis was not the only cause of fractures and that a diagnosis should be confirmed before starting on long-term treatment.

NICE asked the National Osteoporosis Society (NOS) for comments and, in February 2004, announced that it was splitting its appraisal into two. The first looking at recommendations for people who have already broken a bone due to osteoporosis (secondary prevention) and the second to look at the best treatment for those at high risk of fracture but who have not already broken a bone (primary prevention). In those guidelines there is still a restriction on the new drug Forsteo (teriparatide), saying it should only be given to those women over 65 who have not responded to other treatments and have a T score of -4.0 or below from the DEXA scan.

The second section of these guidelines (primary prevention) has now been postponed for further consultation. The hesitation is that the majority of research with osteoporosis drugs has been done on women who have already had at least one fracture. There is not a great deal of evidence to show that these drugs are effective for women below the age of 60 and with no previous fracture. NICE, acting as a government body, has to know that the financial cost is worth it.

Chapter 5

The Nutritional Approach to Healthy Bones

The food that you eat has a significant effect on your bones because the body uses the nutrients from your diet to rebuild and renew them. Certain foods are beneficial for your bones whilst others are not, and it is very important to know which is which – there's much, much more to it than just drinking milk!

Everyone can benefit from an eating plan that concentrates on foods and supplements to boost bone health, but it is equally as important to avoid those substances that can weaken your bones. Much of the information you will read about bone health and osteoporosis concentrates on getting minerals like calcium into your bones, but if your diet is leaching the body of its calcium stores it won't matter how much you ingest through food or supplements – you will be fighting a losing battle.

A popular health message is that calcium-rich foods or calcium supplements will help to prevent osteoporosis, which is true, up to a point. Ninety-nine per cent of the body's calcium is certainly stored in the bones. Bone is a living, hard yet flexible tissue made up of small crystals of calcium, phosphorus and other minerals held together by collagen. The crystals give our bones strength and the bones need constant supplies of calcium for renewal. But there is more to it than that. If you take in too much calcium in your diet your body will not be able to use it all and will merely excrete it in your urine. We do have to keep replenishing our calcium supplies – but we must also make sure we are not depleting our stores of calcium unnecessarily at the same time.

So, before we look at what you should eat for good bone health and which supplements to take (see chapter 6), let's look at what causes the leaching effect on your bones and what you can do about it. In chapter 11, you will find meal plans and recipes to help boost your bone health.

THE ACID FACTOR

One of calcium's roles in the body is to act as a neutraliser – when you eat too much acid food your body calls up calcium reserves from your bones in the form of bicarbonate, an alkaline substance, to counteract the acidity. Therefore, if your diet is highly acidic – high in meat, for instance – it could be causing a leaching effect on your bones. So even if you are eating a calcium-rich diet and taking calcium supplements, if your diet is acidic, you could be losing more calcium than you are gaining.

As you get older your body's ability to excrete acid declines,[1] so you actually become significantly more acidic as time goes on. This is especially important for women around the menopause, who are at greater risk of developing osteoporosis, and therefore need to make their diet more alkaline to counteract this and ultimately protect their bones.

The aim then is make your diet more alkaline by taking a close look at what you are eating and drinking. One of the most highly acid-forming substances which cause most calcium to be leached from your bones is protein, particularly in red meat.

Protein

Protein, in moderation, forms a vital part of the diet because it is the basic building block for all the cells and bones as well as hair, skin and nails. It is made from 25 amino acids, eight of which are called 'essential' because they must be obtained from food, unlike the other 17 which are made naturally by the body.

But protein causes an acidic reaction in the body which calcium then acts to neutralise. The body corrects the imbalance using calcium from the bones and teeth, and once the job is done, the calcium is then eliminated from the body through the urine.[2]

So where does this leave the increasingly popular high-protein diets claiming to help with weight loss – how do they affect the bones? Over the last 80 years many studies have shown that a high protein intake increases the excretion of calcium through urine. It is thought that at protein levels of 175g per day (roughly equivalent to two sausages and a portion of chicken) for every 50g consumed over and above that (another two slices of turkey) you lose an extra 60mg of calcium through the urine.[3] Significantly, for high-protein diet aficionados, proteins in red meat generate more acid than those in fish or poultry.

Unfortunately for bone health, one of the most popular weight-loss diets at the moment is the high-protein diet. It is based on the principle of eating lots of protein, such as meat and eggs, but few carbohydrates. Even fruit intake is strictly limited because of its carbohydrate status. More recently the protein-only diet has been the latest craze to sweep across the US, with a number of celebrities swearing by its ability to promote quick weight loss.

The theory is that sweet and starchy foods make blood sugar levels rise sharply and when insulin is raised, more of your food is converted into fat, and you begin to put on weight. So it is believed that by cutting out anything that prevents a surge of insulin, you will lose weight. It sounds logical, and it can indeed cause dramatic weight loss. However, in the long term, this type of diet is not only unhealthy, but potentially dangerous. When the body is starved of carbohydrates it will look for energy in its glycogen stores. Because 4g (0.14oz) of water clings to every gram of glycogen, you can appear to lose a lot of weight very quickly on a low-carb diet. But the immediate weight loss is water, not fat. Only when the glycogen stores are completely depleted does the body start to dissolve fat cells.

A protein-only diet can cause an abnormal metabolic state called 'ketosis'; which happens when insufficient carbohydrate is stored in the liver for the body to use for energy. The body then has to burn fat in order to get energy (hence the weight loss). Ketones accumulate in the blood, causing side effects such as bad breath (there is a fruity odour of acetone on the breath), poorer concentration and memory and mood swings. These same symptoms are experienced in cases of starvation, and in diabetes mellitus.

Added to this is the fact that a high-protein diet causes a build-up of nitrogen in the body. Nitrogen is a breakdown product of protein, which is normally and efficiently dealt with by the liver and kidneys, and then excreted through the urine. But when the protein content of the diet is very high, excess nitrogen builds up and can damage the liver and kidneys.

There are far healthier ways to lose weight and these are explained in my book, *Natural Alternatives to Dieting*.

Scientists disagree about most issues, and whether or not a high-protein diet is bad for the bones is no exception. Two recent studies have shown that increasing animal protein from meat, poultry and dairy foods did not cause an increase in bone turnover or calcium excretion.[4] However, both studies were of short duration – one lasted two weeks and the other 12 weeks – and when we look at longer studies, there is a strong association between rate of bone loss and risk of fracture following a high intake of animal protein. One long-term study, which followed women over seven years, found that older women who consumed a high animal-protein diet have more bone loss and a greater risk of hip fractures than women on a lower animal-protein intake.[5] So the overall weight of evidence is saying that yes, too much protein causes calcium to be lost.

Because as you take in more protein than your body needs, your body cannot store it, so the excess amino acids (from the protein) are converted to organic acids that would acidify your blood. But your blood never becomes acidic because as soon as the proteins are converted to organic acids, calcium leaves your bones to neutralise the acid and prevent any change in pH (see page 65).

So, how do we ascertain how much protein is too much? Scientists found that women who ate more than 95g (3$\frac{1}{3}$oz) of animal protein per day (equivalent to two chicken breasts and a small carton of cottage cheese) had a higher risk of forearm fractures than women who ate less than 68g (2 oz) per day. The same is not true of vegetable protein (beans, nuts and seeds) – it seems that with these foods, no matter how much you eat, your risk of fracture never rises.[6]

If there was a group of women in the world who had the lowest incidence of hip fractures and osteoporosis, we would want to know what they were eating to achieve that result. So scientists have looked at women and the incidence of hip fractures in different countries. The highest rate of hip fractures is found in Western countries in which women consume between 60 and 80g of animal protein per day. The lowest incidence occurs in Asian and African populations amongst whom animal protein intakes are much lower. One study which looked at women in 33 countries found that hip fractures were related to the ratio of animal to vegetable protein (in the form of pulses). In the countries where the rate of hip fractures was the lowest (for example Nigeria and China), the women ate a largely vegetarian diet, consuming more vegetable protein than animal protein. In the countries with the highest fracture rates (such as Germany and Norway), the opposite was true.[7] The researchers concluded that the critical determinant of hip fracture risk was the amount of acid in the diet (vegetable foods are rich in organic salts like citrates which are metabolised into bicarbonates and reduce acid production) and that lowering the intake of animal food could help to protect the bones.

Rates of hip fractures around the world compared to protein intake[8]

Country	Hip fracture incidence per 100,000 person years	Animal protein intake (grams per day)	Vegetable protein intake (grams per day)
Group with lowest risk of fracture			
Nigeria	0.8	8.1	40.2
China	2.9	10.7	51.2
New Guinea	3.1	16.3	39.7
Thailand	5.0	14.7	34.3
South Africa	7.7	27.8	45.4
Korea	11.5	16.9	68.6
Singapore	21.6	24.5	30.2
Malaysia	26.6	24.3	32.7
Croatia	33.5	26.1	67.8
Saudi Arabia	47.3	35.0	49.1
Chile	56.8	25.0	44.8

Group with middle risk of fracture

Italy	57.2	52.1	51.9
Holland	60.7	53.3	33.6
Spain	65.1	50.1	44.1
Japan	67.3	44.3	42.5
Hong Kong	69.2	44.0	36.7
Israel	75.5	39.7	51.0
Ireland	76.0	59.6	41.7
France	77.0	74.2	36.7
Finland	93.5	55.7	36.4
Canada	110.3	60.4	34.7
Crete	113.0	53.1	55.9

Group with highest risk of fracture

United Kingdom	116.5	54.4	36.3
Portugal	119.8	40.7	48.9
United States	120.3	70.1	32.9
Australia	124.8	64.7	33.3
Switzerland	129.4	62.6	35.2
New Zealand	139.0	70.6	34.3
Argentina	147.8	68.2	36.9
Denmark	165.1	55.6	30.5
Sweden	172.0	59.9	29.8
Norway	186.7	58.6	34.0
Germany	199.3	62.4	35.3

The table above shows how too much animal protein can increase the risk of hip fracture and that the more vegetable protein you eat, the lower your risk. Countries such as Germany with their high-protein diets have 40 times as many hip fractures as poorer nations like Nigeria. In the study, many of the countries with the lowest hip fracture rates are predominantly inhabited by black and Asian populations. When the data were also analysed to look at Caucasian women only, the results still showed that the higher the animal protein intake, the greater the risk of hip fracture. So this was not a cultural difference but a dietary one.

On the basis of the findings above, it is also interesting – and appropriate – to look at vegetarians in Western countries. Research shows that vegetarians generally have greater bone density in later life, losing bone much more slowly than meat-eaters as they age,[9] and have a lower risk of osteoporosis.[10] But research shows no difference in bone loss rates between vegetarians who also eat dairy foods and eggs and those who do not.[11]

It seems that the amount of vegetable protein in the diet is a good indicator of the total amount of vegetables that are eaten and it is this factor that reduces the risk of osteoporosis not the vegetable protein itself.

Eggs and some dairy products contain high levels of sulphur-containing amino acids which will cause an acid effect on the body and so increase calcium loss through the urine. If eaten in high enough quantities, a diet rich in eggs and dairy can have a similarly negative effect on the bones to one high in meat. Certainly, non-dairy vegetarians have higher bone density than meat-eaters.[12]

DAIRY FOODS – GOOD OR BAD?

Whilst it is certainly true that milk and other dairy products contain high amounts of calcium, it is debateable whether this is the best way for humans to get their dietary calcium. A baby absorbs more calcium from its mother's milk than from cow's milk despite the fact that cow's milk contains four times the amount of calcium. What is crucial is not the amount of calcium you put in your body, but how your body deals with it. Many people believe that our systems were not really designed to cope with cow's milk. We are the only animals that drink milk past the weaning stage and we persist in drinking a type of milk that was designed for a completely different species.

A growing number of people find it difficult to tolerate dairy products and many more have been told to cut down on dairy foods because of the saturated fat content and the link with heart disease. Some people are lactose intolerant which means that they have a deficiency of the enzyme lactase and so cannot digest the lactose (milk sugar) found in dairy foods. It is estimated that 90 per cent of Asians, 70 per cent of blacks and Native Americans and 50 per cent of Hispanics are lactose intolerant compared to 15 per cent of North Europeans.[13]

Other people have problems with the milk protein (casein) in dairy foods, which can aggravate skin conditions such as eczema. Milk has now been linked to ovarian cancer (drinking more than one glass of milk per day could double the risk of developing ovarian cancer). Scientists believe that the lactose in milk could over-stimulate hormone production and encourage tumours.[14]

The fact that an increasing number of cows today are fed antibiotics to speed their growth knocks dairy products even further down the list of 'ideal' foods.

You may well have been told to eat more dairy products to boost calcium levels for your bone health and then found yourself reading articles (or books like this one) claiming that dairy products are animal proteins and as such could be detrimental to your bones. Who do you believe?

One answer might lie in looking at different countries and comparing fracture rates with the amount of dairy products those women are eating. In many cultures around the world milk and dairy produce are rarely eaten. In China, for instance, two thirds of the population do not consume milk or milk products regularly.[15] In the West, 70–75 per cent of dietary calcium comes from dairy products and less than 10 per cent from green leafy vegetables and soy bean products,[16] compared with China, where only 20 per cent of calcium comes from dairy foods and 50 per cent from plants.[17] And amongst the older population in China even less calcium comes from dairy products as they follow a more traditional way of eating, whilst the younger generation have taken to a more Westernised diet which includes more dairy products.

How do these figures relate to bone density and fracture risk?

Post-menopausal Chinese women tend to have lower hip bone density than Caucasian women, but sustain fewer fractures,[18] which indicates that culturally they have a lower bone density but not a high bone turnover (see page 32). This is an extremely important distinction, because the crux of osteoporosis is the high risk of fractures – this is what we are trying to prevent.

Japan is another country where dairy products are not routinely consumed and although Americans drink three times more milk than the Japanese, the American hip fracture rate is 2.5 times higher.[19]

With Westernisation, it seems, comes an increase in dairy and animal protein consumption as well as soft, fizzy drinks (see page 75) and a decrease in traditional foods like soybean products, rice and vegetables. It is interesting to note that when countries introduce more of a Westernised diet the fracture rate goes up. In Hong Kong, for instance, the incidence of hip fracture rate has doubled in the past 20 years.[20]

As you will see on the following pages, calcium is not the most important aspect of bone health, and dairy foods are not the only source of calcium.

The dairy food–acid connection

What is the connection between dairy products and acid? Could it be that your body's attempt to neutralise the high acid content of dairy products is, in fact, causing you to excrete more calcium (through your urine) than you are actually eating?

It is possible to measure whether a food causes an acid or alkaline reaction in different ways and this has created some confusion because the same foods can be acid or alkaline depending on which chart you look at! In one of the more scientific methods, however, foods are classified into acid/alkaline/neutral by measuring the 'ash' – a residue left by the mineral content of a food after it has been digested. Hence, 'acidic' in this context

—— A quick-reference guide to acid/alkaline ash foods ——

Acid Ash	Neutral Ash	Alkaline Ash
Meat	Butter	Most fruits
Chicken/fowl	Milk	Most vegetables
Eggs	Vegetable oil	Millet
Cheese	White sugar	Buckwheat
Prunes	Margarine	Coconut
Grains (wheat, oats, rice)		Almonds
Cranberries		
Plums		
Rhubarb		
Spinach		
Peanuts		
Corn		
Most nuts		
Fish		
Legumes		
Caffeine		

Acid ash foods are those that contain chloride, phosphorus or sulphur – minerals that form acid compounds. (Plums, prunes, cranberries, rhubarb and spinach are also included because they contain either oxalic or benzoic acid, organic acids that are not completely broken down in the body. Caffeine, which is found in both tea and coffee, has been included as the byproducts of the detoxification of caffeine are acidic.)

Alkaline ash foods are those that contain magnesium, calcium, potassium, sodium – minerals that form alkaline compounds.

Neutral ash foods – simple sugars and fats are seen as neutral as they do not contain minerals of either the acid or alkaline category.

describes the effect the food has once it has been digested: it is what the food *becomes* once you have eaten it that is important. So for instance lemons have a pH of 2.5–3.0 which is highly acidic, but the ash they leave is very alkaline at pH 9.

The idea that acid foods could affect the body and the skeleton has been around since the 1920s and over time scientists have been looking at different ways of classifying acid and alkaline foods.

In 1995, a different measurement was suggested which looks at the acid/alkaline *effect* of food on the kidneys (where urine is made). The reaction is measured by a factor called Potential Renal Acid Load (PRAL) which was

Table of PRAL values of different foods (for 100g of each food)[21]

Food Groups	Highly Acid	Acid	Alkaline	Highly Alkaline
Vegetables			Broccoli -1.2	Spinach -14.0
			Carrots -4.9	
			Cauliflower -4.0	
			Onions -1.5	
			Potatoes -4.0	
			Tomatoes -3.1	
Fruit			Apples -2.2	Raisins -21.0
			Bananas -5.5	
			Lemon juice -2.5	
			Oranges -2.7	
Grains		Oats 10.7		
		Rice (brown) 12.5		
		Rice (white) 4.6		
		Wheat flour 6.9		
Dairy Products	Cheddar cheese 26.4	Cottage cheese 8.7		
	Parmesan 34.2	Milk 0.7		
		Yoghurt 1.5		

Food Groups	Highly Acid	Acid	Alkaline	Highly Alkaline
Animal Products	Eggs (yolk) 23.4	Beef 7.8 Chicken 8.7 Cod 7.1 Eggs (white) 1.1 Haddock 6.8 Pork 7.9 Trout 10.8 Turkey 9.9		
Legumes		Lentils 3.5 Peas 1.2	Green beans -3.1 Soya beans -4.7	
Nuts		Peanuts 8.3 Walnuts 6.8	Hazelnuts -2.8	
Drinks		Cola 0.4	Beer -0.2 Coffee -1.4 Red wine -2.4 Tea -0.3 White wine -1.2	
Other Foods		Butter 0.6	Sugar (white) -0.1 Olive oil neutral at 0.0	

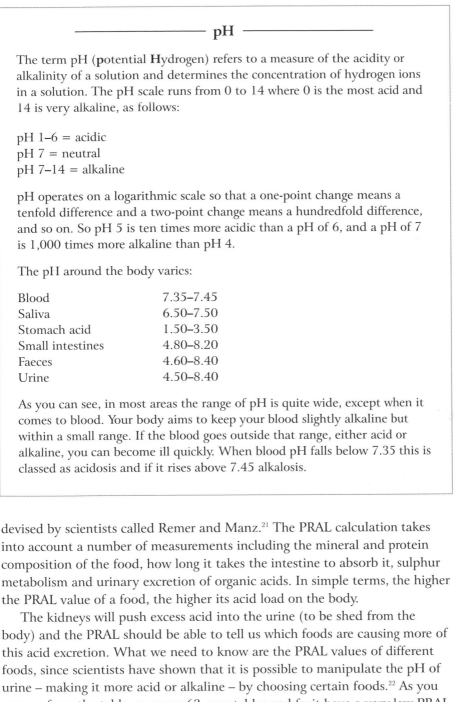

————————— **pH** —————————

The term pH (**p**otential **H**ydrogen) refers to a measure of the acidity or alkalinity of a solution and determines the concentration of hydrogen ions in a solution. The pH scale runs from 0 to 14 where 0 is the most acid and 14 is very alkaline, as follows:

pH 1–6 = acidic
pH 7 = neutral
pH 7–14 = alkaline

pH operates on a logarithmic scale so that a one-point change means a tenfold difference and a two-point change means a hundredfold difference, and so on. So pH 5 is ten times more acidic than a pH of 6, and a pH of 7 is 1,000 times more alkaline than pH 4.

The pH around the body varies:

Blood	7.35–7.45
Saliva	6.50–7.50
Stomach acid	1.50–3.50
Small intestines	4.80–8.20
Faeces	4.60–8.40
Urine	4.50–8.40

As you can see, in most areas the range of pH is quite wide, except when it comes to blood. Your body aims to keep your blood slightly alkaline but within a small range. If the blood goes outside that range, either acid or alkaline, you can become ill quickly. When blood pH falls below 7.35 this is classed as acidosis and if it rises above 7.45 alkalosis.

devised by scientists called Remer and Manz.[21] The PRAL calculation takes into account a number of measurements including the mineral and protein composition of the food, how long it takes the intestine to absorb it, sulphur metabolism and urinary excretion of organic acids. In simple terms, the higher the PRAL value of a food, the higher its acid load on the body.

The kidneys will push excess acid into the urine (to be shed from the body) and the PRAL should be able to tell us which foods are causing more of this acid excretion. What we need to know are the PRAL values of different foods, since scientists have shown that it is possible to manipulate the pH of urine – making it more acid or alkaline – by choosing certain foods.[22] As you can see from the table on pages 63, vegetables and fruit have a very low PRAL and are alkaline. Cheddar cheese has a high PRAL and is more acidic than meat. This means that if you were hoping to protect your bones with large chunks of cheddar, you could be causing the opposite effect. Because of the way your body deals with the acidity of the cheese, you could be losing more calcium than you are taking in from it. Milk is also acidic but not to the same extent as hard cheese – although they are made from the same raw material, milk contains alkalising nutrients that are removed in the process of making hard cheese, the result being that the cheese does not have the alkaline balance.

Although grains like rice have a positive PRAL (acid), countries such as Thailand (where a lot of white rice is eaten) still boast a low rate of hip fractures (see table on page 58) because they eat more vegetable quality foods, only a third of the meat as Westerners and very little, if any, cheese.

So the trends from the table on page 63, show that the negative PRAL values (indicating more alkaline) were found almost exclusively in the vegetable and fruit groups. The highest acid load originated in cheese, followed by meat, fish and grain products. The scientists behind the PRAL system concede that 'similar trends', although with marked deviations for individual foods, were observed by other investigators whose calculations were based on acid-alkaline analyses.[24]

However, it is important that this table is only used as a guide as there are other factors to consider when assessing whether or not a food is beneficial to the health of your bones. Spinach, for example, is strongly alkaline in the PRAL table, yet it should be avoided or kept to a minimum in terms of the prevention and treatment of osteoporosis. This is because it contains oxalic acid which prevents calcium being absorbed in the digestive system – a good enough reason to avoid it! The same applies to coffee and colas: in the PRAL system coffee is mildly alkaline and colas are mildly acidic but both should be avoided for bone health because they interfere with calcium (see pages 71 and 75).

The PRAL values given are also related to the weight of the foods in question. Each value is for 100g of food, but some foods are obviously eaten in larger amounts than others. So, the acid effect of a handful of nuts, for example, will be less than that of a portion of meat.

We also know that legumes and grains which are acidic on the PRAL table contain high levels of potassium (which is alkaline). This makes them extremely useful at helping to promote the retention of bone minerals.[25]

It is thought that fruit and vegetables, even though they are alkaline, can work in another way to stop bone loss independently of their alkaline nature[26] and it is also important to remember that the PRAL values have been calculated assuming that salt does not make any difference to calcium balance, but it does by causing more excretion of calcium through urine.[27] This reinforces the idea that the PRAL table should only be used as a guide.

———————————— **Eating the alkaline way** ————————————

The best way to make your diet more alkaline is simply to aim to have more alkaline-forming foods each day than acid. It has been suggested that the ratio should be 80 per cent alkaline to 20 per cent acid. That is the ideal, but even 70/30 would be good enough. Rather than memorising or constantly referring to tables of PRAL values, which are only a guide anyway, here are some practical suggestions:

- The 80/20 guide does not have to be followed at every meal, but if you have mainly protein in one meal, try to balance this with more alkaline foods in your other meals. When the weather is colder, the ratio might be near 65/35 because you are going to need more warming foods. Just keep in mind your overall aim to eat more alkaline than acid foods in any given day so that the majority of your food on a regular basis is more alkaline.
- Choose good-quality animal protein like fish or eggs (eggs are classed as animal not dairy products).
- Limit the amount of dairy foods, especially cheese, and think about choosing live, organic yoghurt instead.
- If you are having milk, use organic; this contains more Omega 3 essential fatty acids than non-organic milk because the cows are fed differently (although with organic skimmed and semi-skimmed milk the benefit is less, because some of the fat, including the Omega 3 fats, has been removed).
- Choose grains like millet (which is the most alkaline of the grains) and also quinoa for variety and eat beans and vegetables with them.
- And a quick reminder: acid-forming foods are meat, dairy, eggs, fish, shellfish, nuts, grains, beans, soft fizzy drinks, alcohol, tea, coffee and most drugs; alkaline-forming foods are fruit and vegetables.

How to make all this easy

We know it is important to eat a more alkaline diet. Women who consume the most acid-producing diets have four times as many hip fractures as those whose diets are the least acid-producing.[28] We also know that if women are given a strong alkaline substance it dramatically changes how much calcium they lose in a short space of time: when healthy post-menopausal women were given potassium bicarbonate (baking soda) in the form of tablets for two and a half weeks they lost 27 per cent less calcium in their urine and lowered one of the bone turnover markers.[29] That reduction in calcium loss saved them losing about 55mg of calcium per day, which does not seem a big deal. But if that loss continued at that rate for over a couple of decades, that is equivalent to almost half a kilogram or one half of the average woman's skeletal calcium.

——————— Opposites ———————

The idea of two opposites, in this case acid and alkaline, is a major part of many Eastern philosophies and also Traditional Chinese Medicine including acupuncture. The two opposites are termed yin and yang and represent all the opposite principles one finds in the universe. Yang incorporates principles such as maleness, the sun, creation, heat, light and dominance, whilst yin takes in femaleness, the moon, completion, cold and darkness. This principle of opposites also includes the concept that nothing is yin or yang on its own, it is always relative to something else. So we say that one object is dark because we contrast it with another object that is light, and the same for temperature. Ten degrees is hotter than zero degrees but colder than 20. The same goes for acid and alkaline: each food is only more acid or more alkaline than another food it is compared with so everything we eat and drink is on a continuum between acid and alkaline. It is beyond the scope of this book to go into the Eastern traditions, but some examples of the breakdown of food into yin/yang and acid/alkaline include sugar as being yin acid, meat and eggs as yang acid, green leafy vegetables as yin alkaline and root vegetables as yang alkaline.

But there is more. We also know that eating a more alkaline diet has other far-reaching positive effects on your health. It has been suggested that virtually all degenerative diseases are associated with excess acidity in the body including arthritis, heart disease, kidney stones and even cancer. To back this up we also know that diets that are high in alkalising fruits and vegetables have been shown to reduce the risk of breast cancer[30] and heart disease.[31]

Some scientists have suggested that it is unnecessary to focus on more alkaline foods and that by simply taking in extra calcium you will balance the calcium-leaching effect of a high-acid diet. To my mind this makes no sense: it means that your body has to work overtime to buffer excess acid as it really works best when it is slightly alkaline and is going to do everything it can to stay that way. Make the whole process of living as easy as possible by eating alkaline foods which your body does not have to neutralise or buffer.

Can you test for acid/alkaline?

Given the importance of avoiding becoming too acidic (acidosis) it would be useful to have some sort of measure of whether or not you are.

It is no good testing blood because the body keeps the pH of the blood in such a tight range that you would be ill if the pH goes outside that range. There are test strips on the market which indicate the pH of your urine or saliva, but how valuable are they? Are they testing what we think they are testing (i.e. whether our diet is too acid/alkaline)? And is it better to test saliva or urine?

Doctors use urine to test for the presence of glucose, blood, protein, ketones, bacteria and pH. The two scientists who calculated the PRAL values (see pages 62–65) for acid/alkaline foods have shown that as more protein is eaten and the acid load is increased, not only does calcium excretion through the urine increase but the urine pH becomes more acidic.[32] So yes, the effect of your diet on acid/alkaline balance can be seen by measuring urine. Urine gives you an indication of how well your body is working to maintain the proper pH of the blood. If the blood becomes too acidic then the kidneys excrete substances to make the blood more alkaline. If the blood becomes too alkaline then again the kidneys come into play to acidify the blood. The pH of the urine is indicating the efforts of your body to regulate blood pH.

———— Calcium content of different foods ————

There are many foods besides dairy products that contain calcium and you can obtain good supplies by consuming a variety of these foods.

Food	Calcium content (in mg per 100g)
Milk	119
Cheddar cheese	721
Egg (yolks)	139
Eggs (whites)	6
Broccoli	48
Tofu	162
Wholemeal flour	80
Brown rice	10
Cod	21
Trout	86
Figs	145
Haddock	42
Chickpeas	49
Miso	65
Hazelnuts	113[32]

- Tinned pilchards and sardines eaten with their bones contain more calcium weight for weight than milk and they are also rich in Omega 3 essential fatty acids.
- 200g (7oz) of cooked kale or 350g (12oz) of cooked broccoli contain the same amount of calcium as 225ml (8fl oz) of milk.

Urine and saliva show two different aspects of body function. Urine shows digestion and excretion and is a reflection of what you have eaten over the last 12 hours. Saliva, however, will react to what you have just eaten. Saliva is in a state of flux so if you put lemon juice in your mouth your saliva will become more alkaline in order to neutralise the acid. Other factors can also affect the pH of saliva including bacteria and other microbes in the mouth, so that saliva pH is not a reliable indicator of what is going on inside the rest of your body. If you do use saliva for testing though, you should do so first thing in the morning, as soon as you get out of bed, before you have eaten or drunk anything. The ideal pH is around 6.8; if it is less than this (more acid) it means that you need to look at your diet and perhaps increase your intake of fruit and vegetables. It might be worth asking yourself whether you are stressed, because stress makes you more acidic.

Although the normal pH range for urine is 4.5–8.4, the ideal range is 6.5–7.5 and usually reflects the pH of body fluids but may also be affected by urinary tract infections. If the pH is less than 6.5 (more acid) this can reflect a state of potassium depletion, which means that you are not eating enough fruit and vegetables (alkaline foods). Ironically though, if your urine is alkaline at 7.5 or higher, it could indicate that you are in a healthy state, or that you are using too many antacids (indigestion tablets), or that you are in a state of acidosis (because your body is using your alkaline reserves to buffer the effects of acidity). In a state of starvation, urine becomes very acidic so the pH falls quite low.

None of these tests is definitive or diagnostic but if you want to test for pH then I would recommend testing urine rather than saliva as it gives a better overall picture of what is happening as food goes through (and out of) your body.

If you have any concerns about the outcome of a urine pH test, you should see your doctor for a complete urine analysis which will take into account other factors besides pH. You may read elsewhere about challenging your body with different foods and monitoring the outcome. I'm not a great fan of this, as I feel there are too many complicating factors to be sure the tests are giving us a definitive answer in terms of pH. You can use urine testing to give you some idea of how acid or alkaline your body is. This will be, to some extent, a reflection of your diet and how your body reacts and copes with the food you eat. But in the main, I feel it is better to concentrate on increasing your consumption of certain foods and decreasing consumption of others (see page 62) to make your diet generally more alkaline.

CAFFEINE

Caffeine is found in many foods and drinks including coffee, tea (black and green), cola drinks, high-energy soft drinks, cocoa, chocolate and some medications such as painkillers. Coffee has the highest amount of caffeine per ounce but some colas and soft drinks are drunk in larger quantities. This means that certain groups – such as young girls – may be consuming large and unhealthy amounts of caffeine per day. There are other problems associated with soft drinks and their effect on bones and these are discussed on page 75.

Caffeine affects the bones in two ways:

* it causes more calcium excretion through the urine which continues for several hours after it has been ingested
* it decreases calcium absorption in the gut.

In the PRAL table (see pages 63–64) caffeine is seen as alkaline, yet it still has a negative effect on your bones. This is because it is a stimulant and as such causes the release of adrenaline, just as if you were under stress; it is this release of adrenaline that causes the calcium problem. Because of its effects on calcium in the body, caffeine clearly does have a negative effect on bone density and fractures,[34] and drinking more than two cups of coffee per day can significantly increase the risk of hip fractures.[35] There is also a significant association between consuming coffee during teenage years and into adulthood and the risk of osteoporosis.[36]

The other problem is that the effect of caffeine on bones seems to get worse as we get older. A study that looked at women aged 65–77 found that those with a high caffeine intake (more than 300m/18oz) per day, equivalent to about 3 cups of coffee) had significantly higher rates of bone loss at the spine than those who had a low intake of caffeine (less than 300mg/18oz per day).[37]

The other interesting aspect of this study is that the scientists analysed the data further and classified the women according to their genetic make-up (genotype). In the group of women with high caffeine intake, those who had a vitamin D receptor polymorphism (which affects the action of vitamin D and can inhibit calcium absorption) had a higher rate of bone loss than those who were also consuming high caffeine but did not have this receptor genotype.

We are all different and, as the saying goes, 'one man's meat is another man's poison', so our genetic make-up can determine whether or not and how different things affect us. The genetic aspect of osteoporosis is discussed further in chapter 8; however, if you do not know your genotype, the message is that you should cut down on caffeine. And if you have a diagnosis of osteoporosis, caffeine should be cut out altogether.

Drinking tea

Tea also contains caffeine but less than coffee. If you really need your 'cuppa', take care to drink it away from mealtimes. Tannin in tea binds to important minerals such as calcium and iron and prevents their absorption in the digestive tract, so leave a gap of at least one hour before or after eating if you are going to have a cup of regular black tea.

There is research to suggest that tea drinkers can have a higher bone density.[38] It is thought that this could be due to the flavonoid content in tea, which has an antioxidant effect. This idea ties in with other theories showing that free radicals – chemically unstable atoms – may cause decreases in bone mineral density,[39] and antioxidants protect us against the effects of these harmful free radicals. However, as black tea can cause fluctuations in blood sugar which can affect your mood, it is preferable to get the antioxidants from fruits and vegetables rather than from tea.

Green tea can be used in moderation as it has stronger antioxidant effects than black tea, but it still contains some caffeine. Try herbal varieties, such as peppermint instead.

Caffeine is addictive and as you cut it out, you may find that you get withdrawal symptoms which can include: headaches, nausea, tiredness and depression. To minimise these effects, which can be quite dramatic, do not suddenly give up caffeine overnight. Cut down gradually, over a period of a few weeks, substituting alternatives for some of your usual drinks. Begin by substituting decaffeinated coffee for half of your total intake per day, then gradually change over to decaffeinated only. Next, slowly eliminate the decaffeinated as well by introducing other drinks, such as herbal teas and grain coffees.

It is advisable, ultimately, to eliminate decaffeinated coffee as well for two reasons: chemicals have to be used to remove the caffeine and also there are other stimulants in coffee such as theobromine and theophylline which are not good for your health. In addition to the negative effects it has on your bones, coffee is also one of the most heavily sprayed plants in the world: high quantities of pesticides are ingested with every cup.

SUGAR

Like caffeine, sugar also causes excess excretion of calcium in the urine[40] and women who have a greater intake of sweets have significantly lower bone mineral density (up to 11 per cent lower).[41] Indeed, it is actually possible to induce osteoporosis in hamsters by feeding them a sugar-laden diet.[42]

It is also known that the amount of sugar you eat can affect your immune system, and compromise your body's ability to fight infection. It has been

---

Recognising sugar

Be wary of food labels that say 'no added sugar'. In order to make sugar content look lower, manufacturers break down the sugars into various forms, although in terms of the effects they all have on our bodies they are very similar. Words ending in '-ose' all refer to sugars:

- Fructose is fruit sugar.
- Glucose is body blood sugar, fast acting.
- Dextrose is sugar from cornstarch, chemically identical to glucose.
- Lactose is milk sugar.
- Maltose is made from starch.
- Sucrose is common table sugar, made from sugar cane or beet.

When you read a food label compare the *total* sugar figures provided.

---

found that sugar detrimentally affects the process called 'phagocytosis', where white blood cells engulf and consume bacteria and foreign substances.[43]

On average, each of us consumes 1kg (¼lb) of sugar per week, and much of this is 'invisible' sugar, hidden in various foods that you would not necessarily think of as 'sweet'. In 1850, the world production of sugar was 1.5 million tons per year; that figure has now risen to an enormous 75 million tons. We are eating 25 times the amount of sugar we ate 200 years ago.[44]

Sugar is just empty calories. It piles on the weight, provides no nutritional value, and has a negative impact on your bones. I would suggest that you cut down sugar drastically, or, ideally, cut it out completely. You should not add it to drinks or foods such as tea, fruit or cereals, and avoid eating obviously sweet foods, such as chocolate.

It is also important to read the labels, as sugar is added to many different foods, including tinned vegetables, soups, yoghurts and even pasta sauces. One fruit yoghurt, for example, can contain up to eight teaspoons of sugar, whilst a 'healthy' muesli bar can contain just as much. Indeed, sugar is added to practically everything as it is an inexpensive bulking agent. Even some toothpastes contain sugar, but as toothpaste is not a 'food', it does not have to appear on the ingredients list.

Also watch out for the probiotic drinks with 'friendly' bacteria that are very popular. They do contain beneficial bacteria which are good for you (see page 82) but they often also contain large amounts of sugar which feeds the negative bacteria and yeasts like candida. The best way round this is to take the beneficial bacteria as a supplement in capsule form.

The only way sugar is acceptable to eat is in its natural form – the whole sugar cane. This is a 'wholefood' with all the right amounts of fibre, but we never eat it like this. It is when sugar is refined that the problems start. Processing and refinement remove the fibre as well as the vitamins, minerals and trace elements. The same is true for white flour. In order to digest these refined foods your body has to use its own vitamins and minerals, so depleting your stores.

In fact, apart from the negative effects that it has on your bones, sugar also makes it more difficult for you to lose weight. Every time you eat, your body has a choice: it can either burn that food as energy or it can store it as fat. Scientists know that if more insulin is released, more of your food will be converted into fat. What's more, if food is actively being converted into fat, any previously stored fat fails to be broken down. So the more sugar you eat, the more insulin your body releases, and the more fat it stores.

Artificial sweeteners

You may be tempted to substitute sugar with artificial sweeteners: don't. This simply introduces an alien chemical into your body which then has to be dealt with, giving your body extra work to do.

Health concerns abound regarding artificial sweeteners and in particular aspartame, the most commonly used one. Take a look at the labels on foods in your kitchen and you will see that aspartame and artificial sweeteners crop up in fizzy drinks, yoghurts, desserts, tinned foods and the full spectrum of convenience foods. A food or drink described as 'low sugar', 'diet' or 'low calorie', will usually contain an artificial sweetener.

It is also often wrongly assumed that artificial sweeteners help to control weight, but studies have shown that people who regularly use artificial sweeteners tend to gain weight because the sweeteners increase their appetite.[45] Aspartame is 180 times sweeter than sugar and can lead to binge eating and weight problems.

Aspartame has also been linked to mood swings and depression because it alters the levels of the brain chemical serotonin.[46] One of the classes of drugs used for depression are SSRIs (Selective Serotonin Reuptake Inhibitors), which are designed to optimise the use of serotonin, which then helps to lift our mood and reduce appetite. Aspartame works in exactly the opposite way.

In America, the Aspartame Toxicity Information Centre (www.holisticmed.com/aspartame) has been set up, largely because of the concerns regarding aspartame and more serious health problems. When digested, aspartame releases methanol and two amino acids, aspartic acid and phenylalanine, into the body. Methanol converts to formaldehyde (formaldehyde, a toxin, is classed in the same groups of drugs as cyanide and arsenic!) and then to formate or formic acid.[47] Amino acids are fundamental constituents of all proteins, and they interact with each other. They are normally ingested in small quantities in proteins, and in combination with other amino acids. In this case, however, aspartic acid and phenylalanine are being ingested on their own, and in much larger quantities. The result is that they can throw the balance of the metabolism of amino acids in the brain.[48] In other words, they affect the way in which your brain uses amino acids.

Symptoms linked to regular consumption of aspartame include: mood swings, memory loss, numbness and tingling, skin problems such as urticaria and rashes, seizures and convulsions, headaches, eye problems, nausea and vomiting and depression.

There are also concerns that aspartame is addictive, and that people who drink a large number (three to four cans) of diet soft drinks every day, or regularly chew sugar-free gum, may experience withdrawal symptoms if they try to stop.

My advice is to avoid any foods or drinks that contain artificial sweeteners. This is not easy, but as you reduce your intake of sugar and artificial sweeteners, your taste buds will adapt. The natural sweetness of foods such as parsnips and sweet potatoes will become evident and much more pleasing. Sweetened, processed foods will begin to taste 'overly sweet'. If you do find that you need a sweetener for some foods, try small amounts of honey, maple syrup, brown rice syrup and barley malt syrup. These are not only healthier alternatives, in that they have some nutritional value, but they are also less likely to cause swings in your blood sugar levels.

SOFT, FIZZY DRINKS

The greatest concern with soft drinks, in my opinion, is their high levels of phosphorus. When phosphorus levels in your blood rise, a message is sent to your brain, telling it that there is not enough calcium. As a result the body draws calcium from your bones and teeth to balance the high levels of phosphorus. If this happens regularly, your bones will begin to weaken.

Most women should reach their peak bone density at 25 and this should then remain stable until the menopause. Many young women and teenagers, however, who over-indulge in soft, fizzy drinks, are storing up trouble for the future. Colas, often a favourite with teenagers, are particularly high in phosphorus because phosphoric acid is added to 'sharpen up' the taste. Diet colas can contain between 27 to 39mg of phosphoric acid per 100ml.

The pH of colas (with phosphoric acid) has been calculated at between 2.8 and 3.2.[49] This is extremely acidic and the kidneys cannot excrete urine with pH this acidic so the body has to neutralise it in some way. It could do this by diluting the cola but it is estimated that it would take an additional 33 litres of urine to dilute a 330ml can of cola,[50] so if there are enough reserves of sodium and potassium (found predominantly in fruits and vegetables) from the diet it uses those, but if not it uses the calcium and magnesium stored in the skeleton.

Soft drinks are a known risk factor for osteoporosis in women of all ages and, worryingly, an increased fracture rate has been found in girls as young as 8 to 16 years old who drink large quantities.[51] Also by giving phosphorus to post-menopausal women at each meal over a period of 12 months, scientists could monitor its effect on the bones.[52] The bone biopsies showed that bone-forming surfaces decreased and bone-resorbing surfaces increased, which indicates that the phosphorus was causing more bone to be broken down than was being rebuilt. It actually increases bone turnover.

For women, it is my belief that the risks inherent in soft, fizzy drinks are not worth taking and it would be preferable to cut them out altogether. Apart from the phosphorus factor, they are also laden with sugar, caffeine, artificial sweeteners and/or other chemicals. In January 2004, the medical journal *Pediatrics* issued a policy statement by the American Academy of Pediatrics regarding concern about soft-drink consumption through vending machines in schools.[53] The fear was not only for bone health but also the additional calories from these drinks causing obesity and weight problems. They point out that high-fructose corn syrup is the principal nutrient in sweetened drinks, and it appears in high doses – equivalent to 10 teaspoons of sugar in a 350ml(12fl oz) can/bottle. In the UK, there are now children as young as 11 or 12 with Type II diabetes (usually triggered around middle age). Also filling up on soft drinks means that young people are less likely to eat sufficient fruit, vegetables and other nutritious foods.

ALCOHOL

Alcohol can have a negative effect on bones by decreasing the activity of the osteoblasts (or bone-building cells)[54] and increasing bone loss and the incidence of fractures.[55] It also acts as a diuretic, causing the leaching of valuable minerals such as calcium and magnesium.

There is no real consensus as to whether moderate alcohol consumption affects bone density. A number of studies have shown little association between drinking moderate amounts of alcohol and bone density, whilst one says that social drinking is connected with higher bone density.[56] However, with heavy consumption of alcohol, there is an increased risk of falling, and if your bones are not good you should avoid this at all costs. Alcohol definitely affects bone metabolism but the studies do not prove an effect on bone density.

But there are plenty of other reasons to keep alcohol to a minimum, not least that it is full of calories, made by the action of yeast on sugar, and provided in the form of a carbohydrate. Just one glass of wine contains about a hundred calories, whilst a pint of beer delivers around two hundred.

Alcohol acts as an anti-nutrient in that it blocks the good effects of our food by depleting the body of vitamins and minerals, especially zinc which is essential for bone health (see page 103). It also compromises liver function. The liver is the body's waste-disposal unit for toxins, waste products, drugs, alcohol and hormones, ensuring their safe elimination from the body. It also plays an important part in activating vitamin D which is needed for good calcium absorption. There is no doubt that you want your liver to be working efficiently.

Your liver deals with oestrogen so it can be eliminated safely from the body. Oestrogen is not one hormone, but a group of three hormones: oestradiol, oestrone and oestriol. Oestrogen is secreted by the ovaries in the form of oestradiol and the liver metabolises oestradiol to oestrone and oestriol. The liver's ability to convert oestradiol (the most carcinogenic oestrogen) efficiently to oestriol is very important because oestriol is the safest and least active form of the hormone.

The liver also performs other important functions that have a bearing on your health. Among its many tasks are the storage and filtration of blood, the secretion of bile and numerous metabolic functions, including the conversion of sugars into glycogen, which is the form in which carbohydrates are stored in your body. It plays a vital part in metabolising fat (breaking it down properly) and it helps to use up fat to produce energy. The liver also helps to optimise thyroid function.

The best approach is to consume alcohol in moderation. Try to save it mainly for the weekend or special occasions, and when you do drink, do not have more than two glasses of wine or beer.

SALT

Salt is sodium chloride, often found in high amounts in processed and convenience foods. Also, no-fat and low-fat foods tend to be high in both salt and sugar. A diet that is high in salt can affect your bones by causing you to lose more calcium through your urine.[57]

In one study, when women were asked to cut their sodium intake to between 1g and 2g per day (equivalent to no more than one teaspoon), their calcium requirements were reduced by 60mg per day.[58] This means that the more sodium there is in your diet, the more calcium you need to correct the balance.

Sodium is a mineral that is closely associated with your body's ability to balance water retention and blood pressure – the higher the level of blood sodium, the higher the blood pressure. Potassium also helps to regulate your water balance and normalise your heart rhythm – the more sodium you consume, the more potassium you need to counteract this effect. Low blood sugar, diuretics and laxatives can all cause potassium loss.

Interesting research has found that women with high blood pressure experience a faster loss of bone minerals,[59] which is to be expected given that

---

Potassium

Potassium is crucial for bone health and helps to stop the loss of calcium through urine.[60] It is found in large quantities in fruit and vegetables. In order to achieve a healthy balance you should:

- reduce substances that cause a loss of potassium, such as alcohol, coffee, sugar, diuretics and laxatives
- increase your intake of fruit and vegetables
- reduce your sodium intake

---

high levels of sodium cause high blood pressure and leaching of calcium from the bones. So if you have high blood pressure, it would be worth having a bone scan to look at the health of your bones.

Table salt (sodium chloride) is a major source of sodium in the body. It is estimated that in the West we consume 10–20 times more than is necessary. Salt is found naturally in all fruits, vegetables and grains so there really is no need to add more. Notwithstanding this, we not only add salt to our food during cooking and at the table, but it is abundant in most convenience and prepared foods including ketchup, salad dressings, burgers, chips, biscuits and pizzas. Still more sodium gets into your body through sodium nitrate, the preservative used in meat and also monosodium glutamate (MSG), a flavour enhancer, used extensively in convenience and Chinese food.

The current recommendation in the UK from the Scientific Advisory Committee on Nutrition 2003 is to reduce our salt intake from 9g (2 teaspoons) to 6g per day (1 teaspoon = 2.4g sodium) and the Foods Standard Agency 2003 is working with the food industry to reduce the salt levels in processed foods. There is also, however, a lot that you can do to help yourself.

— Recommendations for reducing your sodium intake —

- eat more freshly prepared foods (so that you know the ingredients)
- use salt sparingly and choose sea salt or rock salt as chemicals are added to table salt to make it flow freely
- use herbs, garlic, ginger, lemon juice, tamari (wheat-free soya sauce) and miso in cooking to add flavour
- avoid convenience or prepared foods with a high salt content
- read all food labels carefully

BRAN

Much attention has been given to the role of fibre in the diet in recent years, and the focus has been on adding bran to a poor diet to increase its fibre content. This, however, is ironic, since bran is actually a refined food: it is contained in the grains of cereal plants and then stripped away to be sold on its own. It also contains substances called 'phytates' which bind to valuable minerals like calcium, zinc and magnesium, essential for bone and general health. In other words, they attract these minerals, a bit like a magnet, excreting them, with the bran, from the digestive tract.

If you normally use bran on breakfast cereal for problems with constipation, linseeds (flaxseeds) can be an excellent substitute. Soak a tablespoon of linseeds in water and scatter them over your cereal. For your bowels the seeds are best left whole (they pass out in the same form they go in), so they act like roughage, although if you grind them or buy flax (linseed meal), this allows the body to absorb their nutrients better. Linseeds are rich in phytoestrogens and it is estimated that one tablespoon of linseeds is equivalent to one portion of soya.

SPINACH AND RHUBARB

Spinach and rhubarb, although alkaline vegetables, contain a substance called oxalic acid, which reacts with calcium in the digestive system and stops it from being absorbed. In order to protect your bones I would suggest that you use these foods sparingly. Other leafy greens such as broccoli or spring greens will provide you with the benefits of a green vegetable without affecting calcium absorption.

Aluminium cookware

Aluminium is a heavy toxic metal that can enter your food through cooking utensils and interfere with the body's ability to metabolise calcium. The same applies to aluminium foil and containers. Try to use cast-iron, enamel, glass and stainless-steel cookware and also avoid coated cookware such as non-stick pans which are believed to be carcinogenic.

Antacids or indigestion medication also contain aluminium. The aluminium binds to minerals as it does with aluminium going in from cookware and renders them useless. Indigestion medication aims to reduce stomach acid, but a good level of stomach acid is, in fact, critical for effective absorption of the minerals from your food (see page 107). So instead of taking medication to reduce the symptoms of indigestion, it is far better to address the cause of the problem.

—————————————————— Stress ——————————

Stress is bad for your bones

Our modern lifestyle creates endless stress through traffic jams, late trains, missed appointments, financial worries, work and family. Adrenaline is the hormone that most of us associate with stress. This hormone is released in 'fight or flight' situations and has a powerful effect on the body: your heart speeds up and the arteries tighten to raise blood pressure and your liver immediately releases emergency stores of glucose into the bloodstream to give you instant energy to fight or run. Because it is not necessary for immediate survival, your digestion shuts down. The clotting ability of your blood is also increased, to help prepare your body in the event of injury. This all means that you have been made ready to run faster, fight back and generally react faster than normal.

All this happens very quickly and it should, theoretically, last for only a short time – just long enough to get you out of danger. However, whereas in a life-threatening situation you would take some action, say run or fight, the stresses of modern life are different, and, in a traffic jam, for example, you just sit there and seethe. So what should be a short-lived reaction can go on for extended periods. Whilst you are 'stressed', your digestion will have shut down so that when you are trying to eat, you will get little nutritional value from your food. Most importantly, perhaps, your risk of heart attack and stroke increases dramatically as your blood begins to clot. Your immune system can also be compromised – if you are under stress it will not work efficiently, making you more susceptible to infections which, when they strike, are more difficult to shake off.

Your adrenal glands are responsible for pumping out adrenaline in response to stress or when blood sugar levels are low. But these glands do much more than this. Situated above the kidneys, they are made up of two parts: the medulla and the cortex. It is the medulla that produces adrenaline, whilst the cortex, which is stimulated by hormones from the pituitary gland, produces three kinds of

FOODS THAT HAVE A POSITIVE EFFECT ON YOUR BONES

Like all living tissue, bones need adequate nutrition for proper growth, so it is important that you eat a wide variety of foods in order to get a good supply of nutrients for bone health. Some foods are more beneficial than others for your bones, so let's take a look now at what you should include in your diet to help to feed your bones!

Fruit and vegetables

Most people know that eating fruit and vegetables is good for general health, and recent campaigns have made it well known that we should all try to consume five portions of these per day.

hormones: cortisol, aldosterone (a hormone that acts on the kidneys to regulate water balance) and the sex hormones, oestrogen and testosterone.

Cortisol is a glucocorticoid, and glucocorticoid drug therapy (a steroid used as an anti-inflammatory) is a known risk factor for osteoporosis. Higher levels of cortisol cause increased bone resorption and decreased bone formation. More bone is resorbed because the cortisol interferes with the action of vitamin D in the digestive system and in turn blocks the absorption of calcium. There will be less bone formation because cortisol stops the osteoblasts (bone-building cells) from doing their job. Another critical point about cortisol is that it can suppress normal functioning of the ovaries, which in turn leads to decreased hormone production from the ovaries and over time can stop the menstrual cycle.

Cortisol levels do not even have to be abnormally high for this negative effect on bone to happen; even levels on the higher end of the 'normal' range have been associated with increased fracture risk in older adults.[61]

However, cortisol also has many beneficial roles in the body: it helps to control fat, protein and carbohydrate metabolism, and, in turn, helps energy production, thyroid hormone production and the strength of the immune system. Cortisol is produced at different levels during the day and this rhythm is as important as the amount of cortisol that your adrenals are producing. Cortisol should be highest in the morning and lowest at night. It is a logical rhythm, in that it is highest when you are ready for the day ahead and lowest when you are going to bed. Low energy levels can, for example, be caused by an abnormal adrenal rhythm, particularly if you find it difficult to get up in the morning. Other symptoms of abnormal cortisol levels can include depression, nervousness and insomnia.

You can find out if you have an abnormal cortisol level with a simple saliva test (see page 143) – if stress is a problem for you, it is important to reduce the amount of adrenaline released. Also, it would be worth learning some form of relaxation, stress management techniques or meditation.

Fruit and vegetables supply vitamins and minerals, including vital antioxidants that protect us against the effects of harmful free radicals – chemically unstable atoms that can cause all sorts of damage in your body. Pollution, smoking, fried or barbecued food and UV rays from the sun can all trigger free radicals. Oxygen, which is vital for our survival, can also be chemically reactive and can become unstable, resulting in the 'oxidation' of other molecules, which in turn generates free radicals.

Free radicals have now been linked to health problems, including cancer, coronary heart disease and premature ageing. They speed up the ageing process by destroying healthy cells and they can also attack the DNA in the nucleus of a cell, causing cell change (mutation) and cancer. Antioxidants,

Go organic

Try to buy as many organic products as you can. Because the soil in which organic fruit and vegetables has been grown has not been so depleted, organic produce usually contains more valuable nutrients – another bonus for your bones. One of the practices of organic farming involves crop rotation, which ensures that the soil is enriched rather than depleted. Remember that organic produce, such as carrots and potatoes, do not need to be peeled. Most of the nutrients of vegetables and fruits are concentrated just under the skin. Simply scrub them carefully, with water, and prepare as normal.

Out of all the dairy foods, yoghurt is the most beneficial for your health, but only when it contains the culture *Lactobacillus acidophilus*, a natural inhabitant of our gut. This culture (bacteria) is important because it is one of the defences of the immune system, and helps to keep unhealthy bacteria and invaders, such as fungal infections and viruses, at bay. Yoghurts that are 'live' normally mean that this culture is present, but the cartons can be marked in a variety of different ways. 'Bio' usually means 'live' and will contain a culture like *lactobacillus*. When yoghurts are heat-treated they lose their original culture, so you will not benefit from eating them.

If you can, choose organic free-range eggs. Free-range is certainly kinder to animals, but the birds can still be fed on an inappropriate diet, which can include chemicals and antibiotics, amongst other things. Organic hens have a strict dietary regime, which includes no worrying additives.

If your budget is limited and you are unsure of what to prioritise in terms of organic produce, go for organic grains (such as rice, oats and wheat – examples are organic brown rice and porridge oats). Even if this is the only organic part of your diet, it can make a huge difference. Grains are very small and can absorb more pesticides than other foods.

which occur naturally in the food we eat, all afford protection against free radicals. Vitamins A, C and E, plus the minerals selenium and zinc, are all antioxidants. Good sources of these are found in brightly coloured fruits and vegetables, such as carrots and pumpkins, citrus fruits and green leafy vegetables, such as broccoli and cauliflower.

Exciting new research into the effects of fruit and vegetables on the bones gives us even more reasons to eat plenty of them. The findings have come about through looking at the link between acid/alkaline balance and bone health. Instead of looking at the actual nutrients in foods (for example, calcium in dairy foods), researchers have been looking at the effects of the foods themselves. In the last ten years, scientists have been finding that higher consumption of fruit and vegetables has a positive effect on bone health across all ages and both sexes – young girls and boys,[62] pre-menopausal women,[63] peri-menopausal women,[64] post-menopausal women and elderly women and men.[65]

Fruit and vegetables are thought to benefit the bones because of their alkaline effect on the body (the exact opposite effect of eating animal protein which produces an acidic reaction). Because they are alkaline they do not force the skeleton to release calcium and also magnesium in order to buffer (cushion) the effects of excess acid. Your body aims to keep extra-cellular fluid at an alkaline pH of between 7.35 and 7.45 in order to survive. With a predominantly alkaline diet your body does not have to draw on resources in the skeleton to keep the balance right. Research has shown that even a small drop in pH, making the body more acidic, causes a tremendous surge in bone resorption.[66] It is a difficult balance to strike then, and your body will sacrifice certain areas, even as important as the skeleton, to maintain it.

Having said that, it is not healthy to cut out all the acid foods in your diet or you might end up too alkaline. Your body is happiest with a diet that leans more towards the alkaline, but bone health can also suffer if you do not have enough protein,[67] so getting the balance right is crucial. If you aim for an 80 per cent alkaline to 20 per cent acid ratio (see page 67) you will be on the right track.

Cider vinegar

Interesting research has looked at the effects of vinegar in the diet. Although acidic, vinegar can, in fact increase calcium absorption from food. This ties in with the fact that adequate stomach acid is needed to absorb calcium (see page 107).[68]

The cider variety is the most beneficial vinegar in that it helps to balance potassium and so has an alkalising effect on the body and is therefore good for your bone health. This is one of those paradoxes where a food that starts off acidic actually ends up alkaline when digested (see page 61). My recommendation is either to use cider vinegar on your food (in salad dressings, for example), or to take 15ml (1 tablespoon) of cider vinegar and honey in a cupful of warm water up to three times per day.

Phytoestrogens

With the negative aspects of HRT becoming more widely recognised, many women have begun to look at other ways of managing symptoms of the menopause, and increasing interest has come to rest on a group of foods called phytoestrogens (covered in great detail in my book *New Natural Alternatives to HRT*).

This interest was triggered by scientists who were keen to uncover the reasons why the menopause is experienced so differently around the world. For example, up to 85 per cent of Western women will experience hot flushes,[69] compared with only 14 per cent in some Asian countries.[70] Now scientists are asking the same questions about phytoestrogens and bone, as in many of the cultures where osteoporosis and hip fractures are low, the women eat a fair quantity of phytoestrogens.

What are phytoestrogens?

Phytoestrogens are substances that occur naturally in foods, such as beans like soya and chickpeas, but their name is misleading because it implies that these are plant oestrogens ('phyto' meaning plant). In fact, phytoestrogens act more like SERMs (see page 41), the 'designer' HRTs that provide the beneficial effects of oestrogen where needed (in the bones, for example), whilst avoiding any stimulating effects and even acting as an 'anti-oestrogen', in areas where too much oestrogen can be dangerous, such as the breasts and womb. The *European Journal of Obstetrics and Gynaecology* has dubbed phytoestrogens the 'natural SERMs[71]' because of their balancing effect on hormones.

As discussed in chapter 4, there are two kinds of oestrogen receptors in the body: alpha and beta. The alpha receptors are located in the womb, ovaries and breasts and the beta receptors are in the bones, brain and blood vessels as well as the womb, breasts and ovaries. Phytoestrogens have a weak

---

──── **Types of phytoestrogens and where to find them** ────

There are many different types of phytoestrogens but the three that are relevant to our purposes are:

- isoflavones
- lignans
- coumestans.

Isoflavones are found in high concentrations in soya and other legumes such as lentils, chickpeas, kidney beans and aduki beans. They can be further classified into four other types: genistein, daidzein, biochanin A and formmononentin. Chickpeas and lentils contain all four types, whilst soya contains just genistein and daidzein.

Lignans are found in almost all cereals and vegetables, the highest concentrations being in seeds that provide oils, especially linseeds (flax).

Coumestans are found mainly in alfalfa and mung bean sprouts.

oestrogenic activity that can help to ease menopausal symptoms. Like SERMs they block the alpha receptors in the breasts, womb and ovaries, stopping excess stimulation, and have a positive, stimulating effect on the beta receptors in the brain, bone and blood vessels.[72] This helps to explain why in Japan the number of cases of breast cancer is one sixth of that in the West, yet when Japanese women move to the West and adopt a Western diet, their breast cancer rate rises to Western levels.[73]

What are the effects of phytoestrogens on bone health?

We know that the incidence of osteoporosis and hip fracture is significantly lower in Asian populations,[74] and also that high soya consumption is associated with increased bone density.[75]

Soya

For every story claiming health benefits for soya, there is another suggesting that it can damage health. Soya has been the subject of considerable controversy and has been associated with scare stories about genetic modification. Some reports have claimed that soya can cause an underactive thyroid condition, or that it can be at the root of mineral deficiencies, and there has also been concern about aluminium levels in soya, which have linked it to Alzheimer's disease.

The distinction in health terms lies between traditional soya foods, as eaten by Chinese and Japanese cultures, and processed Western-style soya foods. Some manufacturers buy soya isolate powder and make it into soya milk by adding other ingredients; this is not the same as extracting milk from the whole soya bean, particularly if the bean is genetically modified. The only way you can tell the difference is to read the manufacturer's label on the foods you propose to buy – although GM foods are rarely flashed on labelling, currently if a food is labelled organic you can be sure it is not genetically modified.

If the anti-soya press concerns you, remember that soya is now a big industry, particularly in America, where it is used extensively in margarines and salad dressings and to feed animals, amongst other things. Every scientific study is funded, and every sponsor has a vested interest in the results of the studies they pay for. Many sponsors accept and use the process of genetic modification.

In the other camp sit the pharmaceutical giants who stand to lose a lot of money if natural alternatives to HRT and other menopausal drugs are discovered. And do not forget the dairy farmers, who stand to lose their livelihood if we all swap from cow's milk to soya milk. A lot of people have a lot at stake.

What about the quality of the research into soya?

There has been little substantiation of research citing the negative effects of soya. In fact, a press statement issued in September 2000 by the British Nutrition Foundation said: 'Recent media coverage has raised a number of concerns about possible effects of soya products on health including thyroid abnormalities, mineral deficiencies, Alzheimer's disease and effects in women consuming soy products during pregnancy on the unborn child.[76] But there have been few published studies and those that have been conducted have looked at soya's effect on animals not humans. For the time being, these concerns remain speculative and unproven.'

In one study, for instance, the animals were fed large quantities of *raw* soya flour for five years. Why use raw soya flour in tests? No traditional culture eats raw soya. The scientists were trying to study the effect of protease inhibitors on the pancreas. Proteases (including trypsin) are enzymes which dismantle proteins. The pancreas secretes trypsin which enables your body to break down protein in the small intestine. Raw soya contains trypsin inhibitors which could theoretically stop this process from happening. Out of 26 monkeys tested, only one showed even moderate pancreatitis (inflammation of the pancreas).

———— Which phytoestrogens should you eat? ————

I advise moderation in all things. Eat soya products by all means – they are good for you – but eat them along with other phytoestrogens such as chickpeas, lentils and kidney beans.

The following are good sources of health-giving phytoestrogens:
    legumes (including soya, lentils, chickpeas, aduki beans, kidney beans and peas)
    garlic
    celery
    seeds (including linseeds, sesame, pumpkin, poppy, caraway and sunflower)
    grains (such as rice, oats, wheat, barley and rye)
    fruit (particularly apples, plums and cherries)
    vegetables (particularly broccoli, carrots, rhubarb and potatoes)
    sprouts (such as alfalfa and mung bean sprouts)
    some herbs and spices (such as cinnamon, sage, red clover, hops, fennel and parsley)

The above list reads like the natural and unprocessed diet of many traditional cultures. It goes a long way to explaining why some countries are so much better at resisting osteoporosis than others. Many of these are alkaline foods and eating more of them makes the diet more alkaline. This, as we know, has a beneficial effect on the bones.

Traditionally fermented soya foods, such as miso and soya sauce, are relatively free of worrying protease inhibitors. When tofu is made, these inhibitors end up in the soaking fluid (which is then discarded), and not in the curd itself. Soya milk, which is made from whole soya beans, also involves a soaking process and again, the fluid is discarded after this process.

Soya bean or soya isolate?

Most of the confusion and contention lies in the difference between whole soya beans and soya protein isolates (isolated compounds of soya), and the majority of studies – and therefore the arguments – focus on the latter. In other words, it is not whole soya beans that are controversial.

Soya protein isolates are unnatural contrivances, made in a factory. Technicians use an alkaline solution to remove the fibre from the soya bean after which the beans are put into an aluminium tank with an acid wash where they absorb aluminium. These soya protein isolates undergo a number of other chemical treatments, which add nitrates to the end product. Nitrates are another concern, as they are now known to be potent carcinogens (cancer-forming agents).

The 'food' that results, no longer anything like the original soya bean, is an incredibly versatile bulking agent. It is used to make anything from textured vegetable proteins (with added 'chicken' or 'beef' flavours, for example), to flavour enhancers in soups and sauces (as hydrolysed vegetable protein), lecithin (which is used as an emulsifier in products such as mayonnaise), and even infant formulas, children's snacks and some soya milks.

Up to 60 per cent of processed foods contain soya, including bread, biscuits, pizza and baby food and in the majority of cases, the soya used takes the form of soya isolate.

Traditional soya foods enjoyed in the Far East are divided into two primary types: fermented and unfermented. The fermented type includes soya sauce (also tamari), miso, natto and tempeh. (Tempeh is fermented in two days but miso and soya sauce can take many months. The fermentation process aids digestion.) Unfermented soya includes soya milk and tofu.

Eat a variety of these different phytoestrogens, concentrating on beans as they contain the isoflavones which seem to have the most beneficial effects on bones. Beans are easy to use and they are great added to salads, soups and casseroles. Most beans (although not lentils) need to be soaked, sometimes overnight, before cooking, but you can now buy organic cooked beans in tins from good health-food shops and most supermarkets. (For information on how to cook with beans and other phytoestrogens, see my cookbook *Healthy Eating For the Menopause*.)

Phytates

Phytates are present in the bran or husks of *all* grains and legumes including soya. They can block the uptake of essential minerals, such as calcium, magnesium, iron and zinc, which may be seen as a negative quality and therefore a problem. But the action of these phytates may be one of the reasons that soya seems to have a protective effect against cancer. The phytates bind to iron in the intestines and as iron can generate free radicals which are known to cause cancer, the phytates in the soya act as antioxidants.

Muesli is a good example of a phytate-rich food. It should be soaked before being eaten, so that the phytates it contains will not block the uptake of minerals: pour milk, water or juice over muesli and leave it for about 20 minutes before eating.

Can you have too much of a good thing?

There is an abounding myth that when something is good for you, the more you have of it, the healthier you will be. I see this belief illustrated frequently in the field of nutrition, where people tend to believe that extra quantities of herbs or vitamin supplements will enhance their effects. This can be dangerous as very often the effects of a food or supplement are most beneficial at specific doses, beyond which they can have adverse effects.

Not surprisingly, the myth has spread to soya. Once its beneficial effects became clear, people moved in droves to get as much of it as they could. As a result, you can now buy soya in almost every imaginable form. In fact, there are now even snack bars containing nothing more than *raw*, ground soya beans. Soya should not be eaten raw, nor should it be eaten in excessive quantities. When eaten raw, and in excess, soya can have negative effects, for example on thyroid function.

When you eat soya foods, try to have them in their traditional form – as miso, tofu or organic soya milk. These foods are healthy, and they can have a dramatic effect on your health, particularly during the menopause. Avoid the 'gimmicky' soya bars and snacks unless you know they are made from the whole bean, and even then you should ensure that the beans are not raw or genetically modified. If soya foods are genetically modified they can contain fewer phytoestrogens than non-genetically modified ones.[77]

Water

Your body is 70 per cent water and this is involved in every bodily process including digestion, absorption (both critical to get the minerals into your bones) circulation and excretion. Whilst you can survive without food for about five weeks you can live without water for no longer than five days.

Most people do not drink enough water – ideally you should try to drink around six glasses of water per day and these should replace other less healthy drinks. An excellent start to the day is a cup of hot water with a slice of lemon; it is wonderfully refreshing and excellent for the liver.

Nowadays, knowing which water is best to drink is no easy task:

- *Tap water* can be contaminated with any number of impurities and these vary from one area to the next. Arsenic, lead and copper can all occur naturally in tap water and some water can be contaminated by the pipes in which it is carried. Other substances, such as agricultural pesticides and fertilisers, can leach into the water through the ground.
- *Filter water* does not eliminate every single impurity but it does help. You can buy a jug filter where tap water is poured through a filter, but this must be changed regularly to prevent the growth of bacteria. Alternatively a filter can be plumbed in under your sink for the water to flow through. Use the filtered water for washing fruit and vegetables, cooking and hot drinks.
- *Bottled water* has become very popular, but there are many different kinds:
  – *spring water* may have been taken from one or more underground sources and have undergone a range of treatments, such as filtration and blending.
  – *natural mineral water* is bottled in its natural underground state and is completely untreated. It has to come from an officially registered source, conform to purity standards and carry details of its source and mineral analysis on its label.
  – *naturally sparkling water* is natural water bottled from its underground source with enough natural carbon dioxide to make it bubbly.
  – *sparkling (carbonated) water* has had carbon dioxide added during bottling.
  – *flavoured water* has had different fruit flavours added but usually contains sugar or other sweeteners, so should be avoided.

Because many of the mineral/spring waters are alkaline in nature, scientists have looked at what effect they have on bone health. Bicarbonate-rich mineral water has been found to cause a decrease in excretion of calcium.[78] Of course, calcium is also found in mineral waters and the absorption of calcium from these waters is at the same level as absorption of calcium from dairy products.[79] People who were lactose-intolerant absorbed more calcium from mineral water than from milk.[80] So if you are buying bottled buy 'mineral' rather than 'spring' water, and choose one that is slightly more alkaline (with a pH over 7.3).

Soya and the thyroid gland

Some underactive thyroid conditions are caused by a deficiency in iodine in the blood. Iodine is essential for thyroid function, and some foods (termed 'goitrogens') block the uptake of iodine from the blood. Therefore, any food that is a goitrogen will make an underactive thyroid problem worse. Soya is one of those foods, but so are turnips, cabbage, peanuts, pine nuts, Brussels sprouts, broccoli, kale and millet. When eaten raw and in excess, problems can occur. If you are diagnosed with a severe thyroid problem you will normally be told to restrict your intake of these foods.

Chapter 6

It's Not Only About Calcium

When you think of bones, the first supplement that comes to mind is calcium. It's something we're all taught at school – that calcium is vital for the formation of strong bones and teeth. Although it is indeed crucial for healthy bones the focus must not be exclusively on calcium as there is a whole range of nutrients that contribute – together – to great bone health. This chapter will look at all of these and on page 112 you will find information telling you exactly how much of each you need to take.

Although a good, healthy, balanced diet should provide most useful nutrients, I would still recommend that you take supplements of specific vitamins and minerals. It is important to choose a high-quality brand, as good-quality supplements tend to be the ones that your body finds easiest to absorb. When it comes to buying supplements, I always say, you get what you pay for. Capsules (preferably encased in a vegetable shell rather than gelatine) are better than tablets. A capsule tends to be filled only with the essential nutrients, whilst a tablet can include a variety of fillers, binders and bulking agents to hold it together.

CALCIUM

Calcium is essential for bone health and an important mineral in general as it plays a major role in virtually every function of the body. The level of circulating calcium in your blood is so crucial that your body has a fail-safe mechanism, as we have seen in previous chapters, to take calcium from your bones to keep that level constant.

But how much calcium do you need each day? Unfortunately the optimal intake of calcium is the subject of controversy amongst scientists. Ninety-nine per cent of your body's calcium is stored in your skeleton and every day about 200mg is removed from the skeleton, into the blood, and needs to be replaced. To restore this loss you need to consume about 600mg of calcium (your body needs to take in about three times the amount it loses to allow for the fact that calcium is so hard to absorb).

Thus, 600mg per day are needed just to keep the calcium balance stable. But you need to make allowances for the fact that your bones lose more or less calcium depending on whether your diet is acid or alkaline on any given day (see chapter 5), and of course, that your calcium absorption declines as you get older. So what you really need to know is how much calcium you should consume in order not only to replace what you have lost but also to ensure that you are adequately preventing and treating osteoporosis.

How much calcium is too much?

Calcium is classed as an 'essential threshold nutrient'. This means that whilst good levels of calcium are needed for you to reach peak bone density when you are young, and to maintain good bone density in later life, there is a level above which extra calcium is not just wasted, it can actually be harmful. Too much calcium can inhibit the absorption of other minerals such as magnesium, zinc, selenium and iron and increase the risk of developing kidney stones. It is a question of getting the balance right.

In teenagers, if the daily calcium intake is greater than 1,500mg per day, the skeleton becomes saturated with calcium and calcium excretion through the urine starts to rise.[1] In the UK, the suggested daily calcium intake for young girls and boys (aged from 11 to early 20s) is between 700 and 1,000mg per day, whereas in the USA the recommendation is higher, at 1,300 – 1,500mg. The recommended daily intake of calcium for women over the age of 50 in the UK is 700mg, whilst in the USA it is 1,200mg.

The recommended intake relates to the amount of calcium you would get from combining your food and supplements together. So to get a better picture of the size of supplement you need, you have to work out how much calcium you are getting from your food. There are tables that list the calcium content of different foods (see page 69) but if you worked out your calcium intake at every single meal you would spend so much time looking at charts that you would never have time to eat. Besides, food can vary hugely in its mineral content depending on the kind of soil in which it is grown, whether it is organic and how long it has been stored for. So the tables can only ever offer a broad guide.

To confuse matters further, the dosage of calcium given on the label is unlikely to be the amount of calcium that is available for you to absorb. Calcium is found naturally in combination with another substance, for example calcium carbonate, calcium citrate, calcium gluconate or calcium lactate. These are called calcium 'salts' and some are better absorbed than others as explained below, but they also vary in terms of the actual (elemental) calcium they contain. For instance, only 40 per cent of calcium carbonate is actually calcium. So a 1,250mg supplement of calcium carbonate contains only 500mg of actual calcium, whilst a calcium citrate supplement is only 20 per cent calcium. On the other hand, although there is more available calcium in calcium carbonate you'll actually absorb much more calcium from calcium citrate because it is in a more absorbable form.

It is all very confusing, and that is why I have put in a suggested programme of supplements at the end of this chapter – it should give you a clear idea of what you really need.

Calcium does work

The good news is once you get the dose right, calcium supplementation really can reduce the risk of fractures[2] and has a positive effect on bone density.[3] The greatest benefit seems to be in reducing bone loss five years or more after the menopause.[4] If calcium supplements are stopped then any gains in bone density tend to be lost over the next one to two years.[5] Different doses and types of calcium have been used across the various studies. Calcium carbonate in doses of 500, 1,000 and 1,200mg have been used, as well as calcium gluconate 1,000mg, calcium lactate gluconate 1,000mg, calcium citrate malate 500 and 1,000mg. Again, if you look at the recommendations and doses at the end of this chapter you should be able to find the best regime for yourself.

The best way to take calcium in supplement form is in divided doses during the day as this increases absorption. Calcium carbonate should be taken with meals (the activated stomach acid will aid absorption) but calcium citrate does not need stomach acid for digestion and can be taken with or without food. It is also advisable to take one dose at bedtime. This helps to suppress the normal night-time rise in circulating parathyroid hormone (see page 15) which can increase bone resorption during the night and ensures that you wake up with the same bone density you went to sleep with.[6]

How to check your calcium levels

A blood sample will not provide you with a useful measure of your calcium levels as blood calcium concentrations are tightly regulated by the body's ingenious fail-safe mechanism (see page 14) and will only register as abnormal if you are suffering from malnutrition or an overactive parathyroid gland problem. A hair mineral analysis is a better indicator because you can see high calcium turnover in the results (see page 184 for details of how to arrange this type of test). A hair sample might show higher than normal levels of calcium as calcium is literally being leached from the bones and dumped in the hair. You would then need to take extra calcium to replenish your stores and at the same time work on your diet to stop the leaching effect, then retest to make sure that the level is back to normal.

A question was asked in the *American Journal of Clinical Nutrition*: 'Why do populations which consume low-calcium diets have fewer fractures than

—————————— Choosing a calcium supplement ——————————

- Calcium carbonate: this is one of the cheapest forms of calcium. The price may work in its favour, but calcium carbonate (otherwise known as chalk!) is one of the most difficult forms of calcium to absorb, and your digestive system needs to be highly efficient in order to manage it. As you get older, your digestive efficiency diminishes (how many people in their 60s do you know who can eat an evening meal after 8pm and still sleep soundly?). If you have low levels of stomach acid (see page 107), as is the case with many women over the age of 40, you may struggle to absorb even as much as 4 per cent of the calcium from a calcium carbonate supplement. So, if you do opt for a calcium carbonate supplement you should ensure that you are taking a high enough dose to ensure that it you are absorbing enough calcium.
- Calcium citrate: even with poor digestion, you should still be able to absorb 45 per cent of the calcium from this supplement. This is because calcium citrate is almost 30 per cent more absorbable than calcium carbonate.[7]
- Calcium hydroxyapatite: this has been shown to have only 20 per cent absorption[8] and is basically bone meal. Try to avoid supplements containing bone meal, oyster shell or dolomite as they can contain high levels of heavy toxic metals such as lead, arsenic, mercury or cadmium.

Take a good look at your supplements. If it just says 'calcium' in the list of ingredients then it is likely to be calcium carbonate. Most of the calcium supplements available on prescription contain calcium carbonate and often the chewable ones will also contain an artificial sweetener such as aspartame (see page 74) which is best avoided.

To find out whether the supplement you are taking is in a form that is easy to absorb, try the following test: place your supplement in a glass of warm vinegar (this roughly simulates conditions in your gut) and leave it for 30 minutes, stirring occasionally. If the supplement has not completely dissolved after half an hour, then your supplement is probably leaving your body in much the same form that it entered it! My recommendation would be to change the brand.

If you are taking calcium for prevention of osteoporosis, you will probably have to buy the supplement yourself (as opposed to having it prescribed) and my recommendation is to take it in the citrate form. If you have osteoporosis and have been prescribed a calcium supplement as part of your treatment, you need to ask for the 'healthiest' calcium supplement possible, that is one without artificial sweeteners and colourings.

The bone supplement I use in my clinic contains calcium citrate and is called Osteoplus.

Western societies which consume high-calcium diets?[9] For example, in the Gambia in West Africa there is little evidence of osteoporosis and yet most Gambians have a calcium intake of just 300mg per day. This takes us back to the issue of protein intake (see pages 56–60). Gambians typically consume only 40g of protein per day, just 12g of which is from animal sources.[10] The low protein intake means that the diet is generally more alkaline, and therefore the acid load on the body is very low. This, in turn, means that you are less likely to lose calcium (see page 56) and so a high-calcium diet is not required for balance.

All things considered, I believe it is worthwhile taking calcium supplements, in the form of calcium citrate where possible, and in combination with other vitamins and minerals as detailed below.

VITAMIN D

Vitamin D plays a crucial role in the prevention and treatment of osteoporosis since good levels are needed in order to absorb calcium from your food or supplements. In your digestive system, vitamin D is responsible for calcium absorption – it transports calcium across the wall of the intestines and helps to move both calcium and phosphorus into your bones.

Bizarrely, vitamin D is actually not a vitamin. To be classed as a vitamin, a nutrient has to have an essential compound which the body cannot manufacture and so has to derive from food. Vitamin D functions more like a hormone. Whilst we do get some vitamin D from our diet, the most important source is the amount we produce in our skin following exposure to sunlight. On a sunny day, the ultraviolet light in sunshine converts a substance in the skin into a pre-vitamin D which is then changed in the liver and kidneys into the active form – the hormone calcitriol. This works effectively to maintain constant calcium levels in the blood.

Unfortunately, sunscreen can interfere with the production of vitamin D. In my view, sunlight in moderation is fine, as long as you sensibly avoid exposure during the hottest part of the day and do not take exposure to extremes. I am concerned about extreme recommendations to stay out of the sun or to use very strong sunscreens. The US Environmental Protection Agency is now advising that sunlight could be so dangerous we should 'protect ourselves against ultraviolet light whenever we can see our shadow',[11] whilst in Australia, where sun exposure has been campaigned against for years, vitamin D deficiencies are now being recorded in one out of every four people.[12] It is clear that exposure to the sun is necessary for us to produce vitamin D through the skin, and, by extension, for us to protect our bones.

Vitamin D on its own can prevent fractures by up to 25 per cent, especially in the elderly.[13] When vitamin D is taken with calcium the results

---

Benefits of vitamin D

Besides an important role in the prevention and treatment of osteoporosis, good levels of vitamin D have also been shown to have other benefits:

- An association has been found between people who have musculoskeletal pain, such as lower-back pain, and vitamin D deficiency.[14] Findings have shown that when the deficiency is corrected through supplementation, the pain, which can often be non-specific, is eliminated.[15] This effect on muscle function is important because it has been found that vitamin D deficiency increases the risk of falling, especially in older people. If falls can be prevented, then the likelihood of fracture is reduced.
- Vitamin D is made in the skin by a process in which sunlight changes 7-dehydrocholesterol (a substance manufactured in the body from cholesterol) into vitamin D3 (cholecalciferol). So cholesterol is used to make vitamin D. If you are deficient in vitamin D, your liver may respond by producing more cholesterol to be converted into cholecalciferol.

  If you are trying to correct high cholesterol, it would also be worth asking your doctor to check for vitamin D deficiency by assessing the levels of 25-hydroxyvitamin D (25(OH)D) in your blood.
- Researchers have found that vitamin D has cancer-fighting properties that can be used by breast tissue if the body has enough stores of vitamin D.

---

are even better. One study looking at 3,000 women aged between 69 and 106, showed that those taking 1,200mg of calcium plus 800ius vitamin D per day over three years had 32 per cent fewer non-vertebral fractures and 43 per cent fewer hip fractures than those taking the placebo.[16]

If you start supplementing with calcium and vitamin D, however, it is important to keep going: the combination does help to increase bone density, but if supplements are stopped the effect can be reversed within two years, with bone turnover rates swiftly returning to their original levels.[17]

Vitamin D in the diet

The major sources of vitamin D in the diet are eggs and oily fish. Other sources include fortified foods such as margarines and breakfast cereals. However, there is concern that most people today get only a third of their recommended daily amount from their diet. Scientists have also noted a rise in the disease rickets in children who are not eating enough vitamin D-rich foods and who spend little time outdoors (sitting in front of television or computer screens indoors instead).

Choosing a vitamin D supplement

When selecting a vitamin D supplement, choose one in which the form of vitamin D is D3–cholecalciferol. There is another form – D2–ergocalciferol – but this is not as efficient as D3 in helping to correct low levels or deficiencies of vitamin D in the body.[18]

MAGNESIUM

After calcium, magnesium is the most abundant mineral in your bones, with 60 per cent of the body's magnesium being found in your skeleton. It is as important as calcium in the prevention and treatment of osteoporosis, yet so often is not even mentioned or contained in 'bone' supplements.

Magnesium helps to metabolise calcium and vitamin C, and to convert vitamin D into the active form needed to ensure efficient absorption of calcium. It is also essential for normal function of the parathyroid gland which releases parathyroid hormone – one of the important 'bone hormones'.

Magnesium also helps to regulate the heart rhythm and is involved in the production of insulin (people with diabetes are often low in magnesium).[19] Deficiencies of magnesium have also been linked to high blood pressure and heart disease.[20]

There is little doubt that good levels of magnesium are important for your bone health, whatever your age. There is a recognised association between magnesium intake and bone density in pre-menopausal women,[21] and magnesium is also important for bone growth and development in pre-adolescent girls.[22]

Often, women assume that if they have osteoporosis they must be deficient in calcium. One study compared different groups of women, some with osteoporosis, some post-menopausal but with no osteoporosis and some on HRT.[23] It was found that whilst none of the women in any group had low levels of calcium, the women with osteoporosis had low levels of other bone nutrients, including magnesium and zinc. They also had low levels of the enzyme alkaline phosphatase, an indication that the bone is not renewing itself adequately. The body needs magnesium to sustain normal levels of this enzyme.

A lack of magnesium can cause slow bone growth, decrease osteoblastic (bone-building) activity, increase osteoclastic (bone-dissolving) activity and contribute to fragile bones.[24] It has been observed that on a magnesium-restricted diet rats have started to show abnormal bone turnover.[25]

Long-term use (over two years) of magnesium supplements in post-menopausal women has been shown to prevent fractures, with 71 per cent of the women significantly increasing their bone density and 16 per cent halting bone loss completely.[26]

Magnesium also seems to act as 'nature's tranquilliser': it works to relax muscles and because of this can be helpful in easing cramps and migraines. During a migraine attack the blood vessels around the brain constrict (shut down) and then dilate (open). It is thought that this dilation is the cause of migraine pain and that a magnesium deficiency could increase the risk of subsequent dilation (magnesium deficiency has been found to cause blood vessels to go into spasms). A study in which magnesium was given to migraine sufferers found that not only did it help to ease the intensity of the attacks, it also reduced the duration.[27]

A magnesium deficiency can be tested by blood and for magnesium it is more accurate to look at the red blood cells, rather than the serum (the liquid left after whole blood has been separated into its solid and liquid parts), which is the normal procedure. Another good way to test for a magnesium deficiency is to do a hair mineral analysis and then other minerals such as calcium, zinc, selenium can be assessed at the same time.

Magnesium in the diet

Good sources of dietary magnesium include dark green vegetables, apples, seeds, nuts, figs and lemons.

Choosing a magnesium supplement

Magnesium supplements, like calcium, should be in the most absorbable forms possible. For bone health, my recommendation is to take magnesium as magnesium citrate as citrates are easy to absorb because they require little acidification and so are not so dependent on you having a good digestive system. Avoid chlorides, sulphates, carbonates and oxides since they are not so easily assimilated and may pass through the body without being absorbed.

VITAMIN C

Vitamin C is vital in the manufacture of collagen, a sort of 'cement' that holds the bone matrix (the architecture of the bone) together. Collagen makes up 90 per cent of the bone matrix, so vitamin C is an important nutrient in the prevention of osteoporosis. Scurvy – the disease caused by vitamin C deficiency – is, in fact, a collagen disorder. Less common today than it was amongst sailors who used to spend months out at sea with no access to fresh fruit and vegetables, scurvy is characterised by swollen, bleeding gums followed by the opening of previously healed wounds. Collagen helps with the growth and repair of cells, gums, blood vessels and teeth, as well as bones, and prevents problems like easy bruising because it helps to strengthen blood vessels.

Vitamin C in the diet

Because your body cannot make or store vitamin C you have to get it from your diet, so it is important that you are getting enough of it from what you eat. Good sources of dietary vitamin C include fruits (particularly citrus), green leafy vegetables such as broccoli, cauliflower, berries, potatoes and sweet potatoes.

If osteoporosis is a risk factor for you then I would suggest that you also take vitamin C in supplement form.

Choosing a vitamin C supplement

When buying vitamin C supplements, it is better to buy them as the ascorbate form, such as magnesium or calcium ascorbate as this is a buffered (non-acidic) form of vitamin C and is gentler on the stomach than ascorbic acid – the most common form of vitamin C. It is also better to avoid vitamin C in the form of ascorbic acid because you simply do not need the extra acidity; you should be aiming to make your body more alkaline for the sake of your bones.

THE B VITAMINS

The B vitamins, in general, are important for bone health – it has been found that people whose diets are low in B vitamins are more prone to fractures[28] – and low levels of B12 in particular are associated with more rapid bone loss in the hip.[29]

Folic acid is one of the important B vitamins, and, along with vitamins B6 and B12, it helps to control a substance called homocysteine. This is a toxic by-product of the breakdown of methionine – one of the essential amino acids. It should, under normal circumstances, be detoxified (broken down and excreted) by the body. However, increased levels of homocysteine can be created by a high-protein diet (as protein contains methionine) and then the body requires more of the B vitamins in order to detoxify it.

Two recent studies have shown that an increased homocysteine level is a strong and independent risk factor for osteoporotic fractures (almost doubling the risk).[30] It seems that high levels of homocysteine destabilise bone strength by causing a disturbance in collagen cross-linking in bone. These collagen cross-links are important for the stability and strength of the collagen network and if adversely affected can alter the bone matrix to result in fragile bones.

Homocysteine has also been linked to an increased risk of heart disease because it can cause thickening and hardening of the artery walls, making the blood more likely to clot, damaging the blood vessels and contributing to a build-up of fatty deposits or plaque. It has also been linked to Alzheimer's disease.

The link between homocysteine and heart disease was discovered through a rare metabolic disorder called homocystinuria which causes high levels of homocysteine. Researchers found that children who died from this disorder usually died of blood clots and heart attacks, with their arteries looking like those found in older people. Homocystinuria is accompanied by the early onset of osteoporosis, so scientists have been looking at whether the level of homocysteine, which can be detected through a blood test, could be used as a marker to predict the risk of osteoporosis. The answer seems to be a definite yes.

It is definitely worth having a blood test for homocysteine. (You may have to do this privately as it is not always available on the NHS.) An accurate reading should come from a fresh blood sample from a vein, rather than a fingerprick test. There seems to be some controversy regarding the fingerprick test as, according to the laboratories I have spoken to, when the finger is pricked, then squeezed to release a drop of blood, the cells are also squeezed; red cells can easily rupture, releasing the cell contents – and homocysteine – into the serum, potentially giving a false reading. The good news is that if your homocysteine levels are found to be high, your toxic level can be lowered by taking vitamins.

Folic acid in the diet

Good food sources of folic acid include green leafy vegetables, peas, beans and whole grains like oats and brown rice. These should be increased generally regardless of whether you have a high homocysteine level or not.

Choosing B vitamin supplements

If you have a high homocysteine level then you need to take these doses of B vitamins every day, until the level goes back to normal:

Folic acid	0.5–5mg
Vitamin B6	25–50mg
Vitamin B12	500mcg

If your homocysteine levels are normal, then taking a good multivitamin and mineral with folic acid, vitamin B6 and B12 included will be sufficient. I use one called MenoPlus (see www.naturalhealthpractice.com), for women leading up to and through the menopause, which contains good levels of these vitamins.

When choosing B vitamins, look for vitamin B6 in the form of pyridoxal-5-phosphate (P-5-P). Vitamin B6 can also come as pyridoxine which is harder to absorb. Your body has to convert pyridoxine to P-5-P in order to utilise it and that process is dependent on other nutrients so it bypasses any potential problems if you take it in the biologically active form of pyridoxal-5-phosphate. Even with multivitamins and minerals you are better off getting them with vitamin B6 as P-5-P.

VITAMIN K

Vitamin K is known primarily for its role in helping the blood to clot and was named vitamin K for 'Koagulation'. When you have a cut, proteins are transported to the wound and vitamin K converts these into clotting factors. This stops the bleeding and starts the healing process. If you find that you bruise easily this could be due to a vitamin K deficiency.

Vitamin K is also needed to manufacture osteocalcin, a unique protein found in large amounts in bone. Osteocalcin helps to harden calcium, so vitamin K is vital for bone formation. It is a fat-soluble vitamin and the beneficial bacteria in the gut help to synthesise it. Frequent use of antibiotics can destroy these beneficial bacteria which can lead to a vitamin K deficiency. Women who suffer from coeliac disease, Crohn's disease or ulcerative colitis may also be deficient in this vitamin.

Deficiencies of vitamin K have been linked to fractures due to osteoporosis and low bone density. Women who did not consume enough vitamin K (in one study less than 109mcg per day) had 30 per cent more hip fractures.[31]

Vitamin K in the diet

It is now known that most people in both the UK and the USA are not eating enough vitamin K-rich foods on a daily basis with dietary levels of vitamin K well below recommendations.[32] Good food sources of this vitamin include green vegetables (broccoli, cabbage and lettuce), whole grains and soya. Natto, a Japanese fermented soya bean food, is also a rich source.

Vitamin K supplements

When scientists looked at the daily intake of vitamin K through food and correlated that with bone health, they found that women who were not consuming enough vitamin K through their diet were not eating enough green vegetables (which contain good levels of vitamin K). We know from the previous chapter that vegetables are alkaline and protect the bones, so it is not easy to know from the research whether it is just the lack of vitamin K from the diet that is having a negative effect on bone or a generally poor diet, with low intake of green vegetables. I would think it is probably a combination of both.

The important question then is to know whether taking vitamin K in supplement form has a positive effect on bones. This is a relatively new area of research and good, long-term studies are only just being published. One such study looking at the effects of vitamin K supplementation over three years shows a 43 per cent lower rate of bone loss in the supplemented group.[33] The vitamin K was given in a supplement along with calcium and vitamin D; the addition of vitamin K showed better results than those seen with just calcium and vitamin D together.

The concern with taking vitamin K in supplement form, however, is the risk of blood-clotting problems. It does not seem to lead to an increased risk of thrombosis but it can interfere with anti-coagulant medication (such as warfarin and heparin).

Until further research is available on the long-term safety and effectiveness of taking vitamin K in supplement form, my recommendation would be to increase your intake of green leafy vegetables. This will make your diet more alkaline anyway. If you have taken antibiotics fairly frequently in the past, try taking a probiotic supplement containing good levels of beneficial bacteria so that your body finds it easier to manufacture vitamin K.

The recommended dose of vitamin K in supplement form would be 100–150mcg per day, but eating just one portion of kale will give you 500mcg so it is not that hard to get enough vitamin K from your diet. And you can further increase the absorption of vitamin K from green leafy vegetables by adding oil (in a salad dressing, for example) as vitamin K is fat-soluble, so the oil increases absorption.[34]

BORON

Boron is an important mineral in the context of osteoporosis as it plays a crucial part in the conversion of vitamin D into its active form which, in turn, is necessary for calcium absorption.

Research conducted by the US Department of Agriculture demonstrated that giving post-menopausal women 3mg boron supplements daily resulted in a 44 per cent reduction in the amount of calcium excreted in their urine.[35] The study concluded that boron improved the body's metabolism of both calcium and magnesium.

Boron in the diet

Boron is found naturally in leafy vegetables, fruit, nuts and beans (chickpeas and kidney beans, for example).

Choosing boron supplements

It is useful to take extra boron in supplement form when you are trying to prevent or treat osteoporosis. You can get boron on its own but the easiest and most cost-effective way, is to take it in a combined form with calcium and magnesium. With any supplement programme, the aim is to take the least amount of tablets each day, so having combinations can reduce the number you need to take.

ZINC

Zinc is needed for many different and important processes in the body. There are more than two hundred zinc-dependent enzymes in the system, and zinc is involved in the production of many hormones including thyroid, insulin and sex hormones. It is a useful mineral for appetite control as a deficiency can cause a loss of taste so the tendency is to eat stronger tasting foods with more sugar and more salt. Zinc is vital for the optimal functioning of your immune system. Zinc is also found in higher concentrations in bone than in any other tissue in the body. But how does it help as far as osteoporosis is concerned?

Zinc helps vitamin D to boost calcium absorption from food[36] and, like vitamin C, it is also essential for the formation of collagen.

Zinc is needed for the proper formation of osteoclasts and osteoblasts, the two cells that are essential for renewing bone. Women with osteoporosis have been found to excrete high amounts of zinc through urine, and loss of zinc correlates with more bone loss, so as bone turnover increases, even more zinc is lost.[37]

Zinc is important for bone health before and after the menopause, with research showing that low zinc intake is associated with low bone density in both pre-menopausal[38] and post-menopausal women.[39]

Zinc in the diet

Good dietary sources of zinc are whole grains, pumpkin seeds and fish. Unfortunately, our modern diet tends to be based on a great deal of processed, convenience and refined foods that have been stripped of essential nutrients through the manufacturing process. As a result, 80 per cent of zinc is removed from wheat during the milling process to boost the shelf life of a loaf of bread. So buy good organic wholewheat bread rather than white.

Choosing zinc supplements

As with magnesium and calcium, you want to choose supplements of zinc in their most absorbable form. Choose zinc citrate or zinc ascorbate for maximum absorption and most good multivitamins and minerals will contain zinc so just read the label to check that the zinc is citrate or ascorbate. Try to avoid zinc oxides and sulphates as they are harder to absorb. A zinc deficiency can be tested by blood and also by a hair mineral analysis (see page 141 for more details).

ESSENTIAL FATTY ACIDS (EFAS)

Most people know that the oils we get from nuts, seeds and oily fish (the Omega 6 and Omega 3 essential fatty acids) are vital for good health but they are also important for your bones.

It seems that good levels of Omega 3 fatty acids from oily fish and linseeds can have a positive effect on calcium absorption and bone density.[40] They increase the absorption of calcium from the digestive system and reduce its excretion in urine. They can slow the loss of bone that happens around the menopause,[41] and it has been found that a diet containing adequate amounts of calcium but *not* of essential fatty acids can increase the risk of osteoporosis.[42]

Many of the women I see follow no-fat and low-fat diets and mistakenly believe that anything associated with fat (including oils) is bad for them. Often, they experience symptoms such as dry skin, lifeless hair, cracked nails, fatigue, depression, dry eyes, lack of motivation, aching joints, difficulty in losing weight, forgetfulness and breast pain, as a result – I believe – of this lack of fatty acids.

EFAs 'oil' the body by lubricating the joints, skin and vagina, as well as being a vital component of every human cell. They are also needed to balance hormones, insulate nerve cells, make the skin and arteries supple and to keep the body warm. If a deficiency of essential fatty acids is not corrected, more serious problems such as heart disease, cancer, arthritis and depression can develop.

EFAs in the diet

Essential fatty acids are found in nuts, seeds and oily fish, including herring, salmon, tuna and sardines.

Choosing EFA supplements

Don't be tempted to supplement with cod liver oil capsules. In the sea, fish can accumulate toxins and mercury, which pass through their livers (the organ responsible for detoxification). Extracting the oil from the liver of the fish is likely to provide higher quantities of these toxins than the oil taken from the body of the fish.

If you are vegetarian or prefer not to take fish oil, the other way to get those Omega 3 fatty acids is by taking linseed oil capsules or as a liquid. Linseed oil, also called 'flaxseed oil', contains both Omega 3 and some Omega 6 essential fatty acids.

VITAMIN A

Vitamin A is a fat-soluble vitamin and is stored in the liver. It is an important antioxidant and helps to prevent night blindness as well as playing a crucial role in immune function.

There have been concerns that high levels of vitamin A may have a negative effect on bones and increase the risk of fractures. Vitamin A in the form of retinol, taken as a supplement at levels of between 1,500 and 2,000mcg per day, was shown to decrease bone density and increase the risk of hip fracture in post-menopausal women. Vitamin A taken at a dosage of less than 500mcg per day did not have this effect.

However, in 2004, a study published in *Osteoporosis International* followed over 34,000 post-menopausal women for nine years and stated 'we found little evidence of an increased risk of hip or all fractures with higher intakes of vitamin A',[43] from food and supplements or food alone.

Vitamin A in the diet

Vitamin A as retinol is found in liver, dairy products, fortified margarine and fish oils and it is has been suggested that this could be the one nutrient we may be getting a lot of from just diet alone.[44]

But this does not apply to beta-carotene and the other carotenes. These are found in brightly coloured fruit and vegetables such as carrots, sweet potatoes, apricots, green vegetables, pumpkins, tomatoes, apples and peaches. Beta-carotene can be converted by the body into vitamin A as and when it needs it.

My advice then is that you should still eat foods such as oily fish for their vitamin A content in order to benefit from its positive actions (see above). But I would suggest that you avoid eating liver because the amount of vitamin A stored there will be high. In fact, the liver is also the body's 'waste-disposal unit', as toxins and pollutants pass through it for detoxification, so it is best avoided in any case.

Cod liver oil is extracted from the liver of the fish (and is high in vitamin A), so you'd be better advised opting for fish oil supplements where the oil is extracted from the body of the fish (and the vitamin A concentration is lower).

Choosing vitamin A supplements

Vitamin A is an essential nutrient for eye health, skin and the immune system. Retinol is so called because it is essential for the health of the retina in the eye. Vitamin A is also an important antioxidant which helps to protect cells from damage. For your general and bone health, there will be adequate levels in a good multivitamin and mineral supplement.

Phytoestrogen supplements

In chapter 5, we looked at the benefits for osteoporosis of phytoestrogens (isoflavones), such as soya, in the diet. A review in 2003 looked at the evidence of dietary phytoestrogens and their effects on bone. The researchers, who analysed a large number of different studies, came to the conclusion that 'diets rich in phytoestrogens have bone-sparing effects in the long term, although the magnitude of the effect and the exact mechanism(s) of action are presently elusive or speculative.'[45]

So whilst we know that phytoestrogens in the diet can help to prevent and treat osteoporosis, what about taking phytoestrogens (soya or red clover – both are phytoestrogens) in supplement form? Are these beneficial for the bones?

This is a fairly new area of research in which clinical trials are few and far between and the results not yet conclusive. Research on animals has shown soya isoflavones to reduce bone loss in young rats[46] but not in adult ones.[47]

In humans, most of the studies have been short term – six months or less – which is not very useful when looking at bone health. More recent studies have been slightly longer, and one study carried out over 12 months showed that taking isoflavones such as red clover did not make any difference to bone density, but bone formation markers did increase, suggesting less bone loss.[47] A two-year study looked at the effects of taking soya milk containing 76mg of isoflavones or a placebo soya milk without the isoflavones. The intake of isoflavones over the two years did prevent lumbar spine loss in post-

---

Ipriflavone

This is a synthetic isoflavone which does not exist in nature, but has been engineered to see if it has any beneficial effects on osteoporosis. Results are conflicting. It has been shown to increase bone density[48] and to reduce bone turnover by 29 per cent.[49]

However, in a study conducted over four years, involving 474 women aged 45–75 who were either given ipriflavone at 200mg three times per day or a placebo, no positive effects on bone were seen. Bone density and bone turnover were measured at six-monthly intervals but no difference was found between the placebo or ipriflavone groups for any of the measurements taken. So the ipriflavone did not reduce bone loss or change bone turnover. Thirty-one (or 14 per cent) of the women taking ipriflavone developed lymphocytopenia (a decrease in disease-fighting white blood cells) and for some of them it took two years to get back to normal.[50] Obviously this side effect is a major concern and does outweigh the benefit of taking ipriflavone, especially as it is a synthetic phytoestrogen anyway.

menopausal women but there were no significant changes in the hip.[51] Interestingly, this study also included the effects of applying a progesterone cream and found that the progesterone also had bone-sparing effects, but that when soya milk and progesterone cream were used together the bone loss was greater than with either treatment alone.

In 2004, another piece of research used soya protein isolate with varying amounts of isoflavones in the isolate to see what difference the dose made on bone density. The women, with an average age of 55, were given either 96mg of isoflavones per day, or 52mg or a placebo for 9 months, and then assessed 6 months later. This short-term study showed that no significant positive effects on bone density with any dose of isoflavones. The effect was no different from the placebo.[52]

Putting all this information together it would, I think, be premature to assume that phytoestrogen supplements can prevent or treat osteoporosis. The optimum dose is still not known and none of the trials actually looked at whether phytoestrogen supplements prevent fractures, which is really the most important question.

Remember also that when you consume phytoestrogens naturally through your diet, you are not just eating isoflavones, the food also contains fibre and essential fatty acids. Supplements can rarely match the benefit of the whole food.

DIGESTION AND ABSORPTION

The food that you eat and the supplements that you take are only going to be beneficial if you can absorb their nutrients efficiently. Good levels of stomach acid are needed in order to absorb calcium, and one of the side effects mentioned under calcium carbonate supplements in drug reference books is gastro-intestinal disturbances. This is because they are notoriously difficult to absorb. Calcium, when bound to citric acid, forms bioavailable citrates which are easily assimilated and require little acidification prior to absorption. So calcium citrate supplements are a better choice than calcium carbonate and especially if you have low stomach acid

The stomach is basically a bag full of hydrochloric acid. That's how it is supposed to be. It should have a pH of about 1.5 (extremely acidic) compared to a pH of 7.4 for the blood.

STOMACH ACID HAS THREE MAJOR FUNCTIONS:

- it activates an enzyme called pepsin which digests protein
- it increases the solubility of nutrients (helps them to dissolve) so that they can be absorbed into the bloodstream later on
- it acts as a barrier against infection (bacteria, viruses and yeasts are destroyed by the acid environment of the stomach).

Low levels of stomach acid can result in abnormal intestinal bacteria and bugs, and potentially harmful changes in the levels of beneficial bacteria. Frequent use of antibiotics can cause a reduction in beneficial bacteria, and the right balance of gut flora is required for vitamin K to be synthesised in the digestive system.

Stomach acid also stimulates pancreatic enzymes and triggers bile release into the small intestine. These digest and absorb your food as it passes along the digestive tract and even the best supplements in the world can't help you if your body is not digesting and absorbing properly. You may be eating really well but if you are not absorbing the vital nutrients from your food, this is not good news for your bones or your general health.

A stool sample (which can be tested by post, see page 183) can assess your ability to digest and absorb your food and look at the levels of beneficial and other bacteria and yeasts.

Too little stomach acid

With so many advertisements for antacids on television, radio and in magazines you would think we were all producing far too much stomach acid. The irony is that many people end up taking antacids because they think their digestive systems are *over*-acidic when, in fact, the problem is *under*-acidity Ironically, taking antacid indigestion remedies could be making the situation worse by pulling you into a vicious circle.

Improving your digestion

As you get older your level of stomach acid drops, automatically reducing the efficiency of your digestive system. It is important, therefore, for you to do whatever you can to help it along, and the following tips should prove useful:

- Chew your food well. The first part of digestion takes place in your mouth when food is mixed with saliva containing certain digestive enzymes. Chewing also reduces the size of the food so that as you chew, most of the food comes into contact with these enzymes. Smaller particles of food will also pass more easily through the digestive tract.
- Try to relax when you eat. If you eat when you are under stress, adrenaline automatically shuts down your digestive system (see page 80), so it will be compromised and produce lower levels of stomach acid and digestive enzymes.
- Avoid drinking with food (the occasional glass of wine with dinner is a different matter entirely!). Drinking with food dilutes the digestive enzymes and makes the digestive process less efficient.

─────────────── Testing your stomach acid ───────────────

The following are useful tests you can do yourself to check whether you have too little stomach acid.

- If you suffer with heartburn take one tablespoon of lemon juice. If this helps the heartburn then your stomach acid is low. If the symptoms get worse then you have too much acid.

- Dissolve a level teaspoon of bicarbonate of soda in water and drink it on an empty stomach. If you have enough stomach acid, the bicarbonate of soda will be converted into gas and produce bloating and belching within five to ten minutes. If this does not happen, you are likely to be suffering from low stomach acid.

If, after trying these tests, you suspect that you have low stomach acid it is worth taking a supplement of betaine hydrochloride (plus pepsin) with each meal to see whether it helps the symptoms (see page 113). Steer clear of this, however, if you have been diagnosed with any ulcerative stomach problems or gastritis.

Symptoms of low stomach acid

Low stomach acid can cause the following symptoms:

- bloating – near the end of a meal or up to 30 minutes later
- belching
- heartburn
- a feeling of fullness or food 'sitting' in the stomach
- prominent or dilated blood capillaries around the nose and cheeks
- hair loss in women
- nausea after taking food supplements
- diarrhoea or constipation
- food allergies
- soreness, burning and dryness of the mouth.

HERBS

Black cohosh (*Cimicifuga racemosa*)

Black cohosh is the herb of choice around the menopause because it has been heavily researched and proven effective in terms of controlling symptoms such as hot flushes and night sweats (for more information on controlling menopausal symptoms see my book, *New Natural Alternatives to HRT*).

Now scientists have looked at the herb more closely and are finding that it has positive effects on bone quality too. One study on mice (unfortunately), where their ovaries had been removed, showed that black cohosh slowed down the rate of bone loss with the results similar in magnitude to the group of mice given the SERM drug raloxifene (see page 41).[53]

Black cohosh has also been compared to the oestrogen hormone, oestradiol. In this case rats, again with ovaries removed, were given either black cohosh or oestrogen (as oestradiol) and bone density was measured. The rats given oestradiol showed a profound increase in the weight of the womb, stimulating its size, whereas this negative effect was not seen with the rats consuming black cohosh in the food pellets. The control rats, which were given neither oestrogen nor black cohosh, lost 50 per cent bone density, but this loss was not seen in those given either black cohosh or oestrogen. The researchers concluded that black cohosh 'contains yet unidentified substances with SERM properties which act in the hypothalomo/pituitary unit and in the bone but not in the uterus'. Oestrogen is a builder and stimulates certain tissue to grow, hence the risk with HRT and breast cancer and this situation stimulated the womb (uterus) to grow, but the black cohosh did not. The researchers concluded that black cohosh is acting like a SERM, one of the drugs explained on page 41 that can stimulate bones but does not stimulate the womb or breasts.[54]

The next step is for black cohosh to be used in clinical trials on women with particular emphasis on bone density and fractures. Until we have more information, my recommendation is to use black cohosh to help in controlling any menopausal symptoms but to stick with the supplement programme at the end of this chapter for bone health.

A combination of herbs

Other herbs that can be useful for prevention and treatment of osteoporosis are alfalfa herb (*Medicago sativa*), nettle (*Urtica spp.*) and horsetail (*Equisetum arvense*). These three herbs could be combined and taken together as a herbal tea or tincture.

Nettle tea increases the absorption of minerals, including calcium, and horsetail is a natural source of silicon. Silicon is needed for the growth of bone, skin, hair and ligaments. It is also needed for collagen formation and can inhibit bone resorption and stimulate bone formation.[55] Alfalfa herb contains calcium, but also acts like a phytoestrogen, so helping to stimulate bone growth. It also contains vitamins B5, B6, B12, folic acid, vitamin K and most trace minerals.

HOMEOPATHIC REMEDIES

In homeopathy, different women may be prescribed different remedies for the same problem. Homeopaths take a very detailed history and look not only at the symptoms the person is suffering from, but also their likes and dislikes, whether they are 'hot' or 'cold', their sleeping patterns, emotional factors and much more. The remedy prescribed is then called a 'constitutional remedy' and is unique to that person.

If you want to treat yourself homeopathically, the following remedies can help the body to absorb calcium: calcarea carbonica and calcarea phosphorica.

SUPPLEMENTING YOUR DIET

The aim with any supplement programme is to take the important vitamins, minerals and essential fatty acids via the least possible number of capsules. Many women come into the clinic with a carrier bag full of supplements and ask whether they are taking the right ones and in the right doses, when in fact they are often taking some unnecessary supplements and missing some important ones.

The first rule is that your diet must be the foundation of your health. Food supplements are just what they say – supplementary to your diet. You cannot eat a junk-food diet and hope that supplements will do whatever is necessary for your bones.

Having said all that, nowadays, most of us do not get all the nutrients we need from our food. As a society we eat far too many processed, convenience and refined foods that have been stripped of essential nutrients during the manufacturing process. Furthermore, if you have been dieting over a number of years – either restricting your food intake, or trying different diets, diet drinks or pills – you are more likely than not to be deficient in a number of important vitamins and minerals.

This was confirmed by the National Diet and Nutrition Survey published in 2003 which looked at adults aged 19–64. First of all, only 15 per cent of women and 13 per cent of men achieved the five-a-day target for fruit and vegetables. With vitamins and minerals, 74 per cent of women failed to achieve the Reference Nutrient Intake (RNI – this term replaced the old RDA, Recommended Daily Allowance) for magnesium, 45 per cent for zinc, 84 per cent for folic acid and 15 per cent for vitamin D, which are all important for osteoporosis.

In order for your food to contain the nutrients it needs, the soil in which it was grown needs to be rich in nutrients. Carrots, for instance, will extract the minerals from the soil and you absorb the nutrients when you eat them. But our soil has been overfarmed to the point that it no longer contains all the nutrients we need. Furthermore, pesticides and other chemicals reduce the nutrient content of foods, then we go on to process them, stripping them of even more key nutrients. Extra chemicals put an additional strain on your body, which means that you need *more* key nutrients, but what you are actually getting in your daily diet is *less.*

So, whilst we need to ensure that our eating habits are as good as possible, supplements can make a huge difference to your bone health and in a shorter space of time than diet can alone.

Osteoporosis prevention programme

Normal bone density (T score = 0 to -1)

If your bone density is normal, you can just follow a normal maintenance supplement programme to prevent osteoporosis:

A good multivitamin and mineral supplement, containing calcium and magnesium in the form of citrates, vitamin D3 and also boron – the one I use in my clinic is called MenoPlus. It also contains digestive enzymes to increase absorption

B complex (50mg of each B vitamin per day, *including* the amount you get from your multivitamin and mineral)

Vitamin C with bioflavonoids (1,000mg per day as ascorbate)

Zinc citrate 15mg (*including* the amount you get from your multivitamin and mineral)

Essential fatty acids – either as linseed oil 1,000mg or an Omega 3 supplement containing approximately 300mg EPA and 200mg DHA.

Osteopenia – low bone density (T score =-1 to -2.5)

If you have osteopenia, in addition to the maintenance programme above, you need to add in a good 'bone' supplement.

It is better with a good 'bone' supplement to have more magnesium than calcium because you will get calcium from the multivitamin and mineral supplement and most women are deficient in magnesium rather than calcium:

Calcium citrate	approx. 650mg
Magnesium citrate	approx. 900mg
Vitamin D3	approx. 300ius
Boron	approx. 6mg
Digestive enzymes	
Amylase	approx. 21mg
Protease	approx. 66mg
Lipase	approx. 12mg

The one I use in the clinic is called OsteoPlus.

Osteoporosis (T score less than -2.5)

The aim with osteoporosis is to prevent the problem, but you may only recently have thought about having a scan and found out that your bone density is already in the osteoporotic range. It is important that you have a good discussion with your doctor about the best medication for you and, at the same time, go for a bone turnover test (see page 141). Monitored over a couple of months, this can show whether or not your treatment is working.

You should also follow the dietary suggestions outlined throughout this book, take all the extra vitamins and minerals mentioned above (you will probably only be recommended to take calcium – usually calcium carbonate – and vitamin D) and follow the exercise suggestions in the next chapter. This way you will be using the nutritional approach alongside your treatment to give your body the best possible chance of increasing bone density.

Where to get the right supplements?

There are many good health-food shops and websites around that supply good-quality supplements, but you have to know what to ask for. Some of the better brands are BioCare, Solgar, Viridian and The Natural Health Practice. My supplement of choice for all the different brands is www.naturalhealthpractice.com (01892 507598). I have vetted all the products on this site or given them my 'seal of approval' and they only list the supplements that I recommend in my clinic.

Chapter 7

Take Steps for Stronger Bones

In 2003, the World Health Organisation published an article called 'Exercise interventions: defusing the world's osteoporosis time bomb'.[1] In it they stated that 'modifications to diet and lifestyle can help to prevent osteoporosis and could potentially lead to a significant decrease in fracture rates'.

When it comes to bones and exercise, it is definitely a case of 'use it or lose it'. There is simply no way around this: if you do not continue to make the demands on your bones they will not keep up the bone density.

Nature is very clever – it will not waste energy on functions it does not need, and this applies throughout the human body. If you take laxatives for a long time, for instance, your bowel will often stop bothering to function effectively on its own. Similarly, when astronauts float around in a gravity-free environment in space, there is no need for them to stand up and support themselves, let alone put any stress or pressure on their bones. The result is that within a short space of time their bone density drops (it starts after the first month, so it happens quickly[2]), to the extent that they can lose up to 23 per cent of their bone density during a six-month flight.[3] Astronauts are fit people, so imagine what damage inactivity can do to an older, unfit person with poor diet and no supplementation.

We all need to make exercise a priority, not only for our bones but also for our health in general. During exercise, brain chemicals called endorphins are released, easing the fluctuation of emotions by making you feel happier and calmer. Physical activity is also good for your digestive system as it keeps the bowels working efficiently and also keeps your weight under control by boosting metabolism and burning fat.

We know that being active can bring a 30–50 per cent reduction in heart disease for women.[4] We also know that exercise can reduce the risk of breast cancer: women who exercise routinely for between one and three hours a week have a 30 per cent lower risk of breast cancer, whilst the risk is 58 per cent lower for those who exercise for around four hours a week.[5] Extremes of exercise alter the menstrual cycle dramatically – many women athletes, for instance, do not have periods at all, so it is thought that moderate routine exercise suppresses the production (or overproduction) of hormones, reducing a woman's exposure to oestrogen during her lifetime. Some breast cancers are oestrogen-sensitive, so it makes sense that if the hormone levels are more balanced then the risk of developing breast cancer will be reduced. Further research has shown that the biggest risk reduction in breast cancer is seen when the activity or exercise is later in life – particularly after the menopause.[6] The risk of breast cancer increases with age, so anything you can do to reduce that risk is important, especially as it will help your bones at the same time.

However, in modern society physical activity does not necessarily form a natural part of everyday life. Generations ago, people would walk to work or school, and housework was much more labour-intensive, without all the gadgets we have come to rely on so heavily. Today, however, young children are taken to school by car, school playing fields have been sold off for development and physical education lessons have been pared down in the curriculum. Put this together with the fact that more and more children have a computer and/or a television in their bedrooms and are filling themselves up with fizzy drinks and junk food and it looks as though the osteoporosis epidemic is set to continue, expand, and affect an increasingly younger sector of the population.

———— When to start exercising ————

Exercise is important at any age. Even if you've never exercised before it is never too late to start. Bone will respond and adapt. The only proviso if you have not exercised for a while is to start gradually with gentle exercise. Although your bones need to be stressed to increase bone density, as with everything, you need to apply a little balance. If you stress or strain the bones too much they can break, and the process of building bone strength can put such additional strain on the bones. So take it slowly at first.

If you already have osteopenia or osteoporosis then be careful about certain movements such as forward bending as this can increase the risk of fractures of the spine. Avoid heavy lifting, especially if it is combined with bending forward (as in picking up bags of shopping). Also be careful about twisting as this can cause undue stress on the spine (golf in particular involves twisting movements).

HOW BENEFICIAL IS EXERCISE FOR OSTEOPOROSIS?

In one large study, over 61,000 women, aged 40–77, were monitored over 11 years. The lowest risk of hip fracture was seen in women who were active for at least 24 hours a week (55 per cent lower risk of hip fracture) compared to sedentary women who were active for less than three hours per week. But a significantly lower risk of hip fracture (41 per cent) was seen in women who merely walked for just four hours per week (compared to those who walked for less than one). Even spending a greater part of your day standing was connected with a lower risk, because standing puts demands on the skeleton just to keep you upright.[7]

It is quite clear that not only does exercise prevent bone loss, but research has also shown that it can help to reduce back pain and also to reduce cholesterol levels significantly, by up to 5 per cent.[8]

WHAT KIND OF EXERCISE SHOULD YOU DO?

Although most physical activity is good for your heart, not all exercise is as good for the bones, and some forms of exercise are better than others. The following is a breakdown of various types of exercise and how they can impact on bone health.

Weight-bearing exercise

Your skeleton is constantly fighting against gravity, and it is that fight that helps to maintain bone density. You need to load the skeleton and put it under stress in order for it to respond; it works a little like supply and demand.

Any exercise that is performed against the force of gravity is termed weight-bearing. This can include walking, dancing, jogging, stair climbing, low-impact aerobics, tennis, squash, badminton, skipping and bouncing. Weight-bearing exercise is good for bone density because it forces your bones to lift your weight and fight against gravity. Any exercise that causes the muscles to contract is useful as well because it forces the bone attached to the muscles to adapt and change to the new shape of the muscle.

The important thing is to find a form of exercise that you enjoy. There is no point in starting off with something you hate as you'll never keep it up. Line dancing has become popular in recent years and is great exercise for the bones – particularly if you stamp with gusto. Skipping is excellent too, as long as your bones are not too fragile; and using a re-bounder (a small trampoline) can be very helpful as it is gentle on the joints and yet still provides good weight-bearing exercise.

Swimming is not classified as weight-bearing exercise because you are literally held up by the water – hence it is not considered helpful in the fight against osteoporosis (although it is good for your heart).[9] Aqua aerobics,

---

Walking

Walking is one of the easiest exercises for your bones and also for your general health. The British Heart Foundation says 10,000 steps (about five miles) a day is about the right amount to promote a healthy heart and for good bone health.

Most people only walk around 4,500 steps a day, so for the sake of your bones you need to increase this. The 10,000 steps do not have to be walked all at the same time, so you can split them over the day. Try using a pedometer, a small device worn on your wrist or hip – as well as counting the number of steps you take, it can help to motivate you to walk more. Ways in which you can increase the number of steps you take gradually include walking up the stairs instead of taking the lift or escalator, parking your car further away from the shops or office, getting off the bus one stop earlier and walking the rest of the way or parking the car in the furthest space in the car park when you go to the supermarket. Walking 2,000 extra steps a day takes just 15 minutes so it does not take a lot to make a huge difference.

---

however, are great if they provide resistance against the water (see below), thus improving muscle strength whilst being gentle on the bones and joints for those with established osteoporosis.

Cycling is not weight-bearing either, and there are concerns that over time it can reduce flexibility as it requires such a small range of motion. Rowing, too, is not weight-bearing, and is potentially risky if your technique is incorrect as you will put too much of a strain on your spine, especially if the bone density in your spine is not good. However, if your rowing technique is correct, it could actually strengthen the spine.

Resistance training

Resistance training is the use of weights or bands to provide resistance for your muscles to work against. Muscles exert huge forces on the bone sites to which they attach and as the muscles get stronger through lifting weights, the bones will respond accordingly. If the bones did not respond, they could break – so the body adapts to the demands that are placed upon it.

The best form of resistance training, in terms of beating osteoporosis, is the slow lifting of heavier weights with fewer repetitions and longer rest periods in between.[10] Over time, this technique helps to build muscle which, in turn, increases bone density. Lifting smaller weights quickly and with more repetitions (10–15 lifts between rests) is great for stamina and endurance but does not have the same benefits in terms of osteoporosis.

Resistance training can be performed either in a gym, using machines, or with free weights, like dumb bells or elastic bands.

With machines, the weights are lifted by a lever system which increases (up to tenfold) the effect of the weight.[11] Machines can also isolate muscle groups so that you can load specific bones. This can be useful if you have been told that you have osteopenia or osteoporosis in the hip, for instance, and not the spine, as you can then target certain areas for a greater bone-loading effect. Ask at your local gym or leisure centre for a tour and induction. It is important that you are shown how to use the machines safely, especially if you have established osteoporosis.

The use of free weights has more of a bone-loading effect on the whole skeleton, because it is your body that is controlling the lifting and handling of the weights with no help from a machine. Again, you would be better using these weights under supervision but small dumb bells can be used at home and are helpful for strengthening the wrists (a common fracture site, as there is a tendency to put the arms out first when falling). As when exercising with machines, it is best to start with small weights and increase the load gradually as you get stronger.

You can pick up exercise bands (either like stretchy skipping ropes, or long sheets of flexible rubber) inexpensively at most sports shops. Either work with a personal trainer, or look out for exercise videos that show you the correct technique to use with them. You simply hold one end of the band in your left hand, the other end in your right hand, and pull your hands apart (either over your head, behind your back or out to the sides depending on the muscle groups you are exercising), stretching the bands whilst doing so. As you get stronger you can put your hands closer together on the band, and feel a tougher pull as you exercise.

Yoga, t'ai chi and qi gong

All of these activities can boost bone health because they work the muscles, pull on the tendons attaching the muscles to your bones and stimulate bone growth.

Yoga is a good all-round activity which helps to improve flexibility, suppleness and breathing.

Both t'ai chi and qi gong have mental as well as physical benefits. They improve co-ordination, balance (a number of t'ai chi moves are performed on one leg) and flexibility. A study of t'ai chi participants over the age of 70 showed almost a 50 per cent reduction in the rate of falls within 15 weeks of practising.[12]

Improving balance

Yoga, t'ai chi and qi gong can all help to improve balance. This is an important aspect of bone health, because if you have a tendency to be clumsy or trip over then your risk of fractures can be higher.

There are also some simple exercises you can do to improve your balance:

- Hold on to the back of a strong chair. Stand on one leg for one minute and then change sides. Repeat ten times.

- Hold on to a chair again. Roll on to your toes, count to ten, roll back on your heels, count to ten and repeat ten times.

Once you are finding these two exercises easy to do, try using only one hand to hold on to the chair. When that becomes easy try no hands, then eventually try it with your eyes closed.

Pilates

This is a body-conditioning system created after the First World War by Joseph Pilates, a German nurse and physical therapist, originally to help bedridden patients to recover their muscle strength. Pilates is performed on the floor or on specialised equipment, and has gained widespread popularity over the last decade. The idea is to teach body self-awareness, to strengthen muscles (especially in the back and abdomen) without straining them and to improve flexibility. It is best described, perhaps, as a combination of yoga and weightlifting.

Alexander Technique

This gentle technique was created by a Shakespearean actor called Frederick Alexander in the early 1900s in response to a problem he had with losing his voice during solo recitals. He realised that the problem lay in the way in which he held his head and neck, creating abnormal tensions in certain muscles. Hence, the Alexander Technique is all about unlearning the bad postural habits that create muscle tension and can cause neck and back pain.

The Alexander Technique can improve not only your posture but also your balance, as well as reducing tension and stress in the body. It can also be particularly helpful if your spine is affected by osteoporosis. It is important, however, to find a qualified teacher (see page 183).

--------------------- **Vibrating machines** ---------------------

This is a fairly new approach to exercise and involves standing on a vibrating platform. The idea is that the vibrations trigger the bones to generate electric fields and is based on the theory that electrical charges stimulate bone formation and breakdown. When bones are placed under stress, they bend slightly (become concave) and emit a negative electrical charge; at the same time, the opposite side of the bone which has arched becomes convex and generates a positive electrical charge. These two opposite charges then stimulate the formation of new bone.

Vibrating platforms have been used in studies with Russian astronauts and also on sheep and rats, showing subsequent increases in bone density.[13] They are not yet widely available, however, and further research is needed to look into whether or not they can reduce fractures in people in general.

EXERCISING TOO MUCH

This is probably not a problem for most of us, but it is possible – in theory – to exercise too much. If you over-exercise, your muscles produce lactic acid, which contributes to an over-acidic body. So balance and moderation are the key words.

Intensive training in younger women, say as athletes or ballet dancers, can cause a loss of body fat and often the menstrual cycle can stop. Their high level of activity can mean that they never reach their peak bone density and are at a very high risk of osteoporosis. The high incidence of anorexia in these women leads to amenorrhoea (no periods) and an increased risk of osteoporosis. This cycle is called the 'female athletic triad' and involves three factors: anorexia, amenorrhoea and osteoporosis.

Even if you have passed the menopause, intensive training can reduce body fat, and a build that is too slender could increase the risk of

--------------------- **Exercise and calcium** ---------------------

Exercise and calcium have an interactive effect. As exercise stimulates modelling and remodelling of the bone, the body requires extra calcium to meet this increased demand. So it is important that whilst you increase your physical activity you also make sure you are getting enough calcium and other minerals (see chapter 6).

osteoporosis. It is also important not to overdo it as fat cushions the body, especially around the hips, which is helpful in the event of a fall.

YOUR WEIGHT AND BONE DENSITY

It is not healthy to be overweight and it is a widely recognised fact that obesity increases the risk of heart attacks, high blood pressure, diabetes and more. Yet fat is a manufacturing plant for oestrogen, and it is well known that overweight women have a lower of a risk of osteoporosis, and, conversely, slim women have a higher risk. So, here again, it is a question of balance: it is important that you try to be neither under- nor overweight.

You may feel, as many people do, that you need to diet in order to lose weight. However, the way in which you lose weight has an impact on your bones, and crash dieting, for example, can be critical for your bone health. We know from chapter 6 that essential fatty acids are crucial for bone health, so removing all fat is not a good idea.

One study looked at healthy women aged 44–50 and the effects of lowering fat in their diet and increasing physical activity over 18 months in order to help them lose a small amount of weight and the consequences of this on their bone density. The women ended up with a higher rate of bone density loss at both the hip and spine than those women in the control group who didn't reduce their fat intake or increase their exercise.[14] So even though the women in the study were doing extra exercise, this did not offset the negative effects of losing weight by reducing fat.

Healthy ways to lose weight are discussed in more detail in my book, *Natural Alternatives to Dieting*.

CONCLUSION

Looking at all the research, the good news is that you do not need extreme physical activity to create a bone-building effect, so do not start training for that marathon just yet! Exercise is essential, but do not take it to extremes. The bone remodelling process seems to respond best to change, so try to modify your exercise regime fairly frequently, so that you put varying strains on different parts of the skeleton.

Ultimately, there should be four different elements to your physical activity:

- weight-bearing
- resistance
- balance
- flexibility.

Ensuring that you have a good level of physical activity in your daily life is absolutely critical. And remember that even walking protects your bones, so plan your daily routine accordingly – whatever you do, just get out there and walk!

Chapter 8

Is Osteoporosis in Your Genes?

In August 2000, the Office of Genetics and Disease Prevention in America issued a statement (the Gene-Environment Interaction Fact Sheet) saying: 'Virtually all human diseases result from the interaction of genetic susceptibility and modifiable environmental factors, broadly defined to include infectious chemical, physical, nutritional and behavioural factors. 'Variations in genetic make-up are associated with almost all disease. 'Genetic variations do not cause disease but rather influence a person's susceptibility to environmental factors. 'Genetic information can be used to target interventions.'

What this means is that each of us has a unique set of genes that might make us more susceptible to certain diseases, but understanding the workings of these genes can help us to make diet and lifestyle changes (i.e. changes in our environment) that can reduce our risk of getting these diseases.

So, rather than forcing you to accept life with the spectre of a genetically determined disease hanging over us – the 'oh well, it's genetic, there's nothing I can do about it' philosophy – your genes actually give you important information that you can use to your advantage.

With as much as 85 per cent of your bone density genetically determined,[1] the more you know about the role of genetic factors in the regulation of bone density and your risk of osteoporosis, the better equipped you'll be to deal with it. And crucially, nowhere is the gene–environment interaction more evident than in osteoporosis.

WHAT ARE GENES?

At birth you inherit two sets of genes – one from each of your parents. In 1986 the Human Genome Project was officially started and in 2001 the whole genome sequence was published showing the location of the 30,000 genes that make up the Human Genome, so we now know how many genes the human body has.

Genes contain long, double-stranded segments called DNA (deoxyribonucleic acid). More than 99 per cent of the DNA that makes up our genes is exactly the same in all of us. This means that – despite appearances – we only differ from each other by less than 1 per cent. Chimpanzees share about 98 per cent of our DNA, so we have a lot in common with them as well as with each other.

The 99 per cent of DNA that is the same in all of us determines things like two arms, two legs, heart, lungs and so on, whilst the remaining 1 per cent controls those aspects that make us different from each other, like hair and eye colour. (Identical twins are an exception as they share 100 per cent of their DNA.)

DNA is formed by a sequence of four chemicals (called nucleotides), and it is the arrangement of these four chemicals that gives you your unique genetic code.

Mendelian inheritance is a term used by scientists to describe the inheritance of traits. This is named after Gregor Mendel who discovered in 1865, after breeding 28,000 pea plants, what he called the Laws of Heredity. His research taught us that we receive one set of genes from each of our parents, which means that there are two genes for each trait (like hair colour) that you stand to inherit. One of these is more influential than the other in developing a specific trait. The more powerful gene is said to be dominant and the less influential gene is recessive.

For example, if you receive a gene for brown eyes from your mother and a gene for blue eyes from your father, you are more likely to have brown eyes because the gene for brown eyes is dominant whilst the blue is recessive.

The individual identifying traits or characteristics of each person such as height, blood group or sex are known as their 'phenotype'. You may assume that your phenotype is set at birth, but subtle differences in characteristics between each of us are caused by a combination of genetic make-up (or genotype) and the environment in which you live and develop (see box opposite).

A classic example of this is a man who inherits the gene for being tall (thanks to his genotype), but fails to reach his true height because of malnutrition (thanks to environmental factors that intervened). Thus, the environment can affect the intended working, or 'expression' as it is called, of that gene. The man's phenotype is a combination of both genetic and environmental influences.

However, some characteristics are controlled entirely by inheritance. Your blood group (A, B, AB or O), for instance, is controlled entirely by your genes. Your upbringing has no effect on this. Your sex is also determined by genes. In other species, however, this is not always the case: crocodiles have no sex chromosomes, so when crocodile eggs incubate in sand, low and high temperatures result in female hatchlings, whilst temperatures in the middle range produce males. Environment therefore plays a huge part in this selection.

What are environmental factors?

Geneticists refer to the 'environment' as everything in your surroundings that is not the genotype (genetic make-up). This can include:

- diet
- lifestyle
- culture
- drugs
- chemical exposure
- infections.

As you grow up, develop and live, your genes are washed over by your 'environment' and this interaction can make an enormous difference in terms of your health.

Certain genetic disorders can be passed down through families. Cystic fibrosis is an inherited disorder and the chance of a child getting this disorder depends on whether one or both parents have a particular gene. Sometimes members of a family can carry the gene but not pass on the disorder because the gene is recessive in them.

Other genetic disorders are sex linked because they are caused by genes located on the chromosomes that determine sex. Haemophilia (a disorder in which blood refuses to clot), only affects males. Females can only ever be carriers for the gene.

About 5 per cent of cancers occur because of an inherited gene. It is now known that breast cancer is linked to a gene called BRCA1. But the interesting thing is that having this gene only *predisposes* a woman to breast cancer – it does not mean she is going to get the disease, only that she is more susceptible to it than women who do not have that gene. Japanese women have only one sixth of the rate of breast cancer that women in the West have, yet Japanese women who emigrate to America show an increased risk proportionate to the length of time they have lived there (and have therefore been exposed to the environmental factors that activate that gene). First-generation Japanese women in America have a breast cancer risk similar to that in women who live in Japan, but it is 80 per cent lower than that seen in the third generation (that is grandchildren of the original immigrants).[2] The Japanese women will all have similar genes but when they adopt a Western diet and lifestyle – in other words their 'environment' changes – then their breast cancer rate tends to rise to Western levels.

Osteoporosis is no different. Some women may have a genetic susceptibility to the disease, but if they exercise, eat well and lead a generally healthy lifestyle, the disease simply will not manifest itself.

There is little doubt that the science of genetics answers that age-old question – we truly are a combination of nature *and* nurture.

Faults in the wiring

At one time it was thought that all our characteristics resulted from the Mendelian inheritance. But the science of genetics has come a long way since then; we now have a different understanding based on the fact that although our genes are not modifiable, our environment is, so the blame for many diseases does not necessarily rest solely with our genes.

Genetic disorders are often divided into Mendelian and multifactorial traits. In classical Mendelian inheritance, as we have seen, the colour of your hair is dependent on the genes you inherit from your parents and which is recessive or dominant. In contrast, multifactorial diseases like diabetes, asthma, heart disease and osteoporosis are 'caused by mutations in more than one gene in combination with a contribution from environmental factors'.[3]

So, in those diseases that are classed as multifactorial, such as osteoporosis, where there can be many factors contributing to its cause, changes (mutations) can take place in more than one gene. Whether those genes are 'expressed' or not (and whether you end up getting the disease) depends largely on your environment and your way of life.

The 'mutations' are small variations in the genetic code that have been passed down through generations. Scientists call these variations 'polymorphisms' (meaning 'many shapes'), and it is these changes that make us different from each other. Some polymorphisms are harmless because they occur in the 'non-coding' portion of the DNA, so they don't have an impact on our health. From the Human Genome Project it is now known that at least 50 per cent of our DNA is made up of this 'non-coding' DNA or 'junk' DNA. But other polymorphisms such as cystic fibrosis, muscular dystrophy and sickle cell anaemia are serious.

The most common type of polymorphisms are known as single-nucleotide polymorphisms (SNPs – pronounced 'snips'). A SNP is a change in the DNA sequence that involves a variation in a single nucleotide. Nucleotides are the structural building blocks of DNA (see above).

Polymorphisms occur randomly and some are passed on down the generations if they offer some sort of advantage in certain situations. A good example of this is sickle cell anaemia. People who are carriers for sickle cell anaemia (meaning they have only inherited the defective gene from one parent, and the disease does not manifest itself in them), find that the mutation helps to protect them from malaria. Malaria attacks red blood cells but carriers of sickle cell anaemia have differences in their red blood cells that give them protection. So if you live in Africa and you are a carrier for sickle cell anaemia you'll be at a distinct advantage.

But a polymorphism that may be helpful in one environment might not be so helpful when the environment changes. The genetic make-up of Pima Indians, for instance, allows them to survive for longer than most of us without food. This is known as the 'thrifty genotype'. This 'thrifty gene' was extremely beneficial in times when food supply was uncertain. But these days, with food in abundant supply, the same gene gives the Pima Indians a distinct disadvantage, rendering them more susceptible to obesity and diabetes.

Many SNPs have no effect on our health whilst others can put us more at risk of certain diseases or influence our response to medication.

In the field of osteoporosis, genetic profiling is now being used to identify people who will respond positively to bisphosphonate drugs (like alendronate and risedronate) and those who will not. It can also accurately pinpoint those who are most likely to experience side effects and those who will not – even before they take the medication.[4] This type of profiling has also been used in cancer treatment.

In time, this area of science, termed 'pharmacogenetics', will alter the way in which conventional medicine is practised. In the future, two different people with the same disease but different genetic make-up will be prescribed a completely different drug to treat their condition.[5] Genetic information will be used to match the right drug with the right person. In June 2004, the UK government announced a £50 million investment, designed to make the NHS 'a world leader in genetics-based healthcare' – a huge investment in this area of research and development for the future.

The idea of individuals having different responses to the same disease is evident to all of us in everyday life. One person may have smoked all their life and drunk like a fish but is still skipping around, bursting with health, right into their 80s and 90s. Another person, however, smoking the same number of cigarettes, might die of lung cancer before the age of 45. The person most badly affected did not inherit lung cancer, but probably inherited a susceptibility to environmental influences (in other words they were far more sensitive to smoking). It is this susceptibility that increases or decreases your chances of getting a disease.

So, research is showing that we are all a mixture of genetic make-up and the environment to which our genes are exposed. Before the concept of genotype and phenotype we would have talked about a person's constitution. The man who drank and smoked into his 90s would have been said to have a strong constitution and the one who died at 45 a weak one. Yet we always

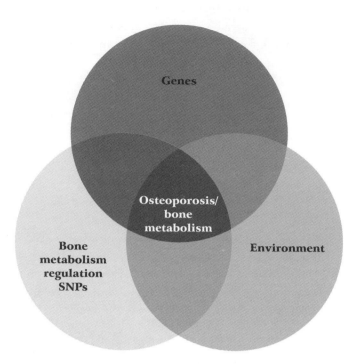

Interaction between genes, environment and SNPs.

recognised the fact that lifestyle factors could have an effect on constitution. It's a cruel fact of life that some people can get away with much more than others simply because of the cards they were dealt at birth.

SNPs are known to play a significant role in the development of many degenerative illnesses such as heart disease and – significantly – osteoporosis. At the moment almost 100,000 SNPs have been identified and over time research will show how these relate to different illnesses.

What are the SNPs for osteoporosis?

If the science of genomics is to be of any use, it is important to be able to identify the polymorphisms that you can work with to make a difference. This means assessing the extent to which intervention in the form of lifestyle changes (diet, food supplements, herbs or drugs) can reduce the risk of developing a disease.

Bone density is considered to be a 'polygenic trait'. This means a number of different genes are responsible for its functioning, and they are called 'candidate genes' – problems with any or all of them could make them 'candidates' for the risk of osteoporosis.

When you take a closer look at the genetic profile of osteoporosis, certain genetically determined factors have been identified as being associated with the risk of developing the disease. These include the way in which your body creates and uses:

- collagen
- calcitonin
- vitamin D
- parathyroid hormone
- inflammation
- oestrogen
- homocysteine
- vitamin K

Collagen

Collagen makes up 90 per cent of the bone matrix (network) and scientists have identified polymorphisms that can lead to abnormal collagen formation. This, in turn, can cause reduced bone mineral density and increased risk of osteoporosis.

The gene called 'Collagen type 1 alpha 1' (COL1A1 for short) is considered to be a genetic marker for bone formation, and polymorphisms in this gene can cause problems with bone synthesis. At the moment, COL1A1 seems to be the most helpful of all the candidate genes for osteoporosis, and research has shown that if you test someone for this gene, it can more accurately predict fractures than bone density scans.[6]

Scientists have found that people who have a specific polymorphism of the COL1A1 gene respond well to increased calcium intake, whilst those who have a different polymorphism of the same gene do not.[7] This refined analysis allows health practitioners to fine-tune their osteoporosis treatments rather than issuing blanket advice to 'take calcium, it's good for your bones'.

It has been suggested that this genetic marker may help to explain why certain cultures have a much lower risk of osteoporosis than others – the polymorphism is common in Caucasian populations, for instance, but rare in Africans and Asians, where the risk of osteoporosis is traditionally much lower.[8]

Calcitonin

Calcium is normally incorporated into the bones by the action of the hormone calcitonin. This hormone regulates calcium metabolism and can decrease blood calcium levels by slowing the activity of osteoclasts (bone-dissolving cells) and stopping bone loss (resorption).

We know that the calcitonin receptor controls the action of calcitonin, and now scientists have found a polymorphism in the calcitonin receptor gene (which they call CALCR). If you have this SNP you could have decreased bone density and an increased fracture risk.[9] A woman who already has osteoporosis and who is identified as having a CALCR polymorphism can have her drug treatment more effectively directed towards calcitonin therapy rather than the more traditional bisphosphonates (see chapter 4).

Vitamin D

Vitamin D plays a major role in bone and calcium metabolism. It regulates the absorption of calcium from the digestive system, bone loss and bone dissolving and the production by osteoblasts (bone-building cells) of the bone-building protein, osteocalcin.

We all have a vitamin D receptor (VDR) gene. Polymorphisms in this gene can inhibit calcium absorption and decrease bone mineralisation, increasing the risk of osteoporosis. Studies have shown that polymorphisms in VDR are associated with decreased bone density in the hip, spine and wrist.[10] They are also linked with increased levels of inactive osteocalcin which indicates a higher bone turnover.[11] Certain VDR polymorphisms have also been linked to a two-fold increase in the risk of hip fracture.[12]

The VDR genotype is the most extensively studied gene in the field of osteoporosis. However, research has thrown up conflicting results. Some research looking at the effects of this polymorphism in relation to osteoporosis found no association between VDR and bone health.[13]

The interesting conclusion that scientists have put forward is that in those studies where there does not seem to be a correlation between VDR and osteoporosis, the intake of calcium and vitamin D that the women in the studies are taking, seems to offset the negative effects of this VDR genotype.[14] This shows again that although a polymorphism may be present, it is possible to reduce its negative effects.

The same conclusion was seen in a study mentioned in chapter 5 which looked at whether or not caffeine increases the risk of osteoporosis. The same quantity of caffeine caused a significantly higher bone loss in women who had the VDR receptor polymorphism than in those who did not.[15] So, the more you know about your genetic make-up, the better equipped you will be to know where you should focus your attention: women with certain VDR polymorphisms, for example, would need to use different strategies, such as good levels of calcium and exercise, to help with osteoporosis rather than increasing vitamin D. (See page 186 for information on how to be tested for the different osteoporosis polymorphisms.)

——————— **Vitamin D receptor and breast cancer** ———————

As well as vitamin D's important role in bone health, it also plays an important part in the immune system and has been studied in relation to cancer, particularly breast cancer.

It is known that breast tissue can use the cancer-fighting properties of vitamin D as long as the body has enough stores of this fat-soluble vitamin. Women who are exposed to sunlight and have a high level of vitamin D at the time of diagnosis of breast cancer seem to have a better prognosis than those whose level is lower.[16]

So what about women who have a vitamin D receptor polymorphism – how does that affect their risk of breast cancer? VDR polymorphisms are associated with breast cancer risk and are also thought to be linked to the actual progression of the disease.[17] But we know from genetic research that a disease is an interaction between genetic make-up and the environment in which genes are expressed, so it should be possible to reduce the risk of that disease developing.

A study in the medical journal *Pharmacogenetics* which looked at VDR gene polymorphisms and the risk of breast cancer concluded that having certain VDR polymorphisms 'may be an important modifier of individual breast cancer risk...especially if they have a positive family history of breast cancer'.[18]

Parathyroid hormone

Polymorphisms in the parathyroid hormone gene can increase parathyroid hormone activity which, in turn, increases bone resorption (loss), and can contribute to decreased bone density and the risk of osteoporosis. The parathyroid hormone receptor (PTHR) regulates the action of parathyroid hormone and so can increase bone resorption.

Inflammation

Genetic marks of inflammation are an interesting area in osteoporosis research. It is easy to link inflammation with joint problems like arthritis but not with bone density and fractures.

Your immune system protects you from invading organisms like bacteria and viruses. In order to function effectively it needs a form of communication to transfer information from one cell or organ to another, and this is accomplished by a group of signal molecules called cytokines (pronounced site-o-kines). These are proteins which stimulate or calm the response of the immune system. They can also cause cells to multiply and divide.

Ideally, there should be a balance between pro-inflammatory and anti-inflammatory cytokines and they should be used appropriately, depending on the situation that demands them. So if you cut yourself, pro-inflammatory cytokines will come into play to activate white blood cells; there will be swelling and redness at the site of the wound, whilst your body mobilises itself to heal the wound and clot any bleeding. Fish oil stimulates the production of anti-inflammatory cytokines, which is why it is helpful in alleviating arthritis (inflammation in the joints).

It is known that one of the pro-inflammatory cytokines (Interleukin-6) stimulates the activity of bone-dissolving cells (osteoclasts). So, if you naturally have higher levels of pro-inflammatory cytokines, your bone breakdown is likely to be higher.[19] IL-1 and TNF-alpha have a strong effect on bone resorption and stop bone formation – not a good thing for building good bone density.

Unfortunately, due to a feedback mechanism in the body, any small increase in the pro-inflammatory cytokines, IL-1 and TNF alpha, will lead to a significant increase in IL-6. Then, IL-1 and TNF alpha are further increased. This means the inflammatory process gets stuck in a vicious circle. But on the positive side, if any one of these three cytokines is absent (perhaps because your body is more balanced and not producing them), then levels of the other two will drop, so decreasing bone loss.[20]

The two most extensively researched cytokine polymorphisms are those connected to IL-6 and TNF-alpha. As would be expected, polymorphisms of the IL-6 gene are connected with a lower bone density and therefore a higher risk of osteoporosis,[21] as are polymorphisms of TNF-alpha.[22]

Types of cytokine

Cytokines can be divided into two categories: pro-inflammatory and anti-inflammatory.

Pro-inflammatory cytokines include:
- Interleukin-1 (IL-1)
- Interleukin-6 (IL-6)
- Interleukin-8 (IL-8)
- Interleukin-12 (IL-12)
- Tumour necrosis factor-alpha (TNF-alpha).

Anti-inflammatory cytokines include:
- Interleukin-4 (IL-4)
- Interleukin-13 (IL-13).

———————— **Cytokines and the menopause** ————————

The menopause is associated with a higher risk of osteoporosis because of the decline in oestrogen around this time. As the ovaries slow down their production of oestrogen, the immune system signals a spontaneous rise in pro-inflammatory cytokines, particularly IL-1, IL-6 and TNF-alpha.[23] So, it could be that the increase in both the number and activity of osteoclasts seen at the menopause may actually be triggered by the immune system.

This may not be too much of a problem if your health is generally good and your immune system is not unduly overworked. But if your basic health is not great, you may experience severe joint pains at the menopause. This could indicate that the pro-inflammatory cytokines are working overtime, causing your joints to become inflamed.

It is important that your immune system functions well. But everything in the body must be balanced – your thyroid, for example, should be neither under- nor over-active, and the same holds true for your immune system. When your immune system becomes too 'active' you can develop auto-immune problems. This means that your body cannot distinguish between its own cells and those that are foreign invaders. So it mounts an immune system attack, only against itself. Rheumatoid arthritis and lupus are two examples of auto-immune diseases and some scientists are suggesting that osteoporosis could also be auto-immune.

Oestrogen

Oestrogen helps to increase bone density so the oestrogen receptor gene is an important candidate gene for osteoporosis.

The new 'designer' HRTs, the SERMs (see page 41) work by stimulating the oestrogen receptors in the bones and not those in the breasts and womb. So drugs are now being designed to target oestrogen receptors specifically. More in-depth knowledge of the oestrogen receptor gene polymorphisms is going to be invaluable for future research.

At the moment, we know that polymorphisms of the oestrogen receptor gene (dubbed ER – from the American 'estrogen') have been found to be related to the onset of the menopause[24] and also to bone density.[25] Polymorphisms in this candidate gene have been shown to determine the risk of fractures independently of the level of bone density.[26]

Homocysteine

In chapter 6 we saw that the breakdown of one of the essential amino acids (methionine) results in a toxic substance called homocysteine, that high levels

————————— **Controlling inflammation** —————————

If you suffer from joint pain, headaches and fatigue, you could have a tendency towards a pro-inflammatory response, and these could be symptoms of general chronic inflammation in the body. If this is the case, you could also be experiencing increased bone loss.

The good news is that nature provides us with substances in the diet that help to control these pro-inflammatory cytokines.

The most important of these are the essential fatty acids. We saw in chapter 6 that essential fatty acids increase the absorption of calcium from the digestive system and reduce excretion of calcium in the urine. But they actually play an even greater part in preventing and treating osteoporosis.

Essential fatty acids fall into two categories – Omega 6 and Omega 3 – and they are termed essential fatty acids because they are, quite simply, essential. We cannot produce them in our bodies so we have to get them from our diet. Years ago we used get a good balance of Omega 3 and Omega 6 oils from our food, but a typical Western diet today contains nearly ten times more Omega 6 (margarines, nuts and seeds) than Omega 3 (oily fish, soya, linseeds) oils, resulting in much higher levels of pro-inflammatory markers.

By increasing your intake of Omega 3 fatty acids you will trigger a decrease in the production of Interleukin-1, Interleukin-6 and tumour necrosis factor-

of homocysteine are a risk factor for osteoporosis and that it can be lowered by taking a combination of B vitamins including B6, B12 and folic acid. The process by which homocysteine is detoxified by the body is called methylation, and is dependent on these B vitamins in order to function properly. High levels of homocysteine in the body generally indicate that it is not being detoxified, usually because of a deficiency of these B vitamins. But in around 40 per cent of people with high homocysteine, the level does not go down even when they increase their intake of B6, B12 and folic acid. These people have a polymorphism that prevents the detoxification of homocysteine. This is a risk factor not only for osteoporosis, but also for heart disease, diabetes and Alzheimer's.

Methylenetetrahydrofolate reductase (MTHFR for short!) is an important enzyme in folic acid (folate) metabolism and polymorphisms in MTHFR lead to high homocysteine levels. It is known that polymorphisms in MTHFR are connected with reduced bone density.[27]

My recommendation would be to have a blood test for homocysteine (see chapter 6 for information about how to go about this) if you have a high risk alpha, which in turn calms the immune system down. The aim is to increase your intake of oily fish and linseed (flax) oil as well as taking supplements if needed. The increase in Omega 3 fatty acids, will show a subsequent decrease in pro-inflammatory cytokines.[28] Whilst a positive change can be achieved through diet alone,[29] my suggestion would be to take supplements of Omega 3 essential fatty acids for three months, alongside working on your diet.

The anti-inflammatory quality of Omega 3 fatty acids makes them a candidate for research into their benefits in rheumatoid arthritis, psoriasis, ulcerative colitis and heart disease. As stated in one of the medical journals: 'many of the placebo-controlled trials of fish oil in chronic inflammatory conditions demonstrate significant benefit…and lowered use of anti-inflammatory drugs.'[30]

As well as making sure you have enough of the Omega 3 essential fatty acids you can also reduce the inflammatory response in your body by cutting out certain foods. We know from chapter 5 that cheese, red meat and poultry are acidic. They contain a substance called 'arachidonic acid', which encourages the production of hormone-like substances called prostaglandins. The prostaglandin that is produced from saturated fats is PGE2, a highly inflammatory substance that can cause swelling and pain and, in some cases, thicken the blood itself. It can also trigger muscle contractions and constriction in blood vessels. The Omega 3 essential fatty acids produce PGE3 prostaglandins which are anti-inflammatory and anti-spasmodic.

of osteoporosis, heart disease or diabetes. If your level is found to be high you should take a good combination of vitamins B6, B12 and folic acid at the dosages outlined on page 100. A follow-up test should be arranged after three months and if your homocysteine level is still high it would be worth having a genetic test for the MTHFR polymorphism (see chapter 6 for information on how to go about this). If this polymorphism shows up, a different combination of food supplements is then needed to overcome the problem – a qualified practitioner can give specific advice as to what is required.

Vitamin K

Vitamin K is an important vitamin in relation to osteoporosis and there is a protein called apolipoprotein E (APOE) which helps to transport it from the intestines to the bones. There are three polymorphisms of APOE: APOE*2, APOE*3 and APOE*4. The APOE*4 variation is associated with increased risk of hip and wrist fractures, independent of the bone density.[31]

APOE*4 is an interesting polymorphism because it is also associated with the risk of developing heart disease and having high cholesterol – high LDL ('bad') cholesterol and low HDL ('good') cholesterol.[32] The polymorphism APOE*4 is found in much higher frequency in indigenous populations (such as Pima Indians, see page 127), amongst whom food supply is frequently scarce.[33] People with an APOE*4 polymorphism will absorb more cholesterol from food as their intestinal absorption of cholesterol is much more efficient and their bodies are programmed to make the most of each fat calorie consumed.[34] This is why the Pima Indians suffer such high rates of obesity and diabetes.

─────────── **Other candidate genes** ───────────

Other candidate genes for osteoporosis are currently being studied:

- transforming growth factor beta-1 (TGFbeta-1) which regulates bone mass
- osteocalcin which is a marker of osteoblast activity
- insulin-like growth factor-1 (IGF-1) which stimulates the growth of the skeleton.

This is a very active field in terms of research; it will be interesting to see how this develops over the next few years.

HOW USEFUL IS GENETIC TESTING?

Think of life and genetic testing in terms of a game of cards. There are some cards you are dealt that cannot be changed, and you are stuck with them for the whole game. Others, however, may not be the best cards you could get, but might be useful depending on how you play them. But if you could not even look at your hand, you would have little chance of winning. So it is with genetic testing – it gives you important information that you may be able to use to your benefit.

In some diseases inherited under the Mendel's Laws of Heredity such as cystic fibrosis, the progression of that disease is inevitable. But, as we have seen, there are genetic diseases that are not inevitable because of multiple gene interactions. Osteoporosis is an excellent case in point. Its gene mutations are modifiable – they can be switched 'on' and 'off' by environmental factors such as lifestyle, diet and toxins. This is known as gene-gene-environment interaction.

So there is clearly value in predictive genomic testing to identify those particular polymorphisms, which we know to be modifiable. Given certain information, we might be able to change the risk of a particular disease by altering lifestyle and diet – the 'environment'.

For osteoporosis there is a number of candidate genes that could be tested (as seen above), but it is important to test for those that have the most clinical relevance in terms of prevention and treatment and also those that are most common.

If you are interested in having a predictive genetic test for osteoporosis then see Appendix 5 on page 186. These predictive genomics tests are particularly relevant for women with a strong family history of osteoporosis. But they can also be useful for women who are proactive about their health and like to work on prevention, rather than waiting for a problem to happen.

Ethical dilemmas

Advances in genetic testing have opened up new doors in the field of prevention and treatment of osteoporosis, and this is an extremely exciting field. However, all aspects of genetic testing are dogged by ethical conflict.

Some people are concerned that because we know so much about genes, in the future embryos could be selected according to those that provide the best genotype, and that one day genetic engineering could actually put certain genes (for intelligence or athletic ability, for example) into embryos. Certainly, pre-implantation genetic diagnosis is now used for IVF treatment where a single cell is removed from the embryo and genetically screened for diseases that may be carried by males and not females. If any are found (haemophilia, for example) the male embryos are then discarded. Genetic screening has also been used to select an embryo that may provide a suitable bone marrow donation for a sibling with a particular disease.

Critics of predictive genomic testing suggest that diet, lifestyle and environment are much more important than genetic make-up in the potential development of disease and that people could end up being treated for illnesses they do not have but are worried they might get. Significantly, they claim, these tests will play on your fears.

I strongly disagree, however. Take a cholesterol test, for example. Although it is not a genetic test, does discovering that your cholesterol levels are high fill you with fear of having a heart attack? High cholesterol does not automatically predict a heart attack – there are many other factors that contribute to heart disease and cholesterol is just one of them. What the test does is to tell you and your doctor that if something is not done about your high cholesterol you could be at increased risk of heart disease. You can then take a more preventative stance.

My aim, through nutritional medicine, has always been to return a patient to good health by addressing the underlying cause of the problem and then to work on prevention. Conventional medicine is certainly excellent for crisis management – if someone is involved in a car accident they want to be taken to hospital for treatment and not be told about the best combination of antioxidants to take. However, in general terms, prevention is rarely a significant goal in conventional medicine.

Conventional medicine tends to focus on treating the symptoms of disease rather than the underlying cause so that when, for example, anti-inflammatory drugs are stopped, the painful joints return because the drugs did not address the reason why the joints were painful in the first place.

Preventative medicine will be the medicine of the future, and predictive genomic testing features largely in this discipline. It gives us vital information about possible risk factors and will increasingly allow conventional medicine to progress so that it can evolve from a one-size-fits-all approach to the right drug for the right person at the right time.

Chapter 9

The Plan of Action
for Osteoporosis

By now you will have read much of the information and advice in this book and – with a bit of luck – you will be feeling inspired to put at least some of into practice. However, after years of working hands-on with patients in my clinic, I know that all the details about tests, diet and supplements can be overwhelming, and it can be very difficult to know where to start. So to make it easier for you to know what to do, this chapter contains a simple step-by-step Plan of Action, I have put together for you to follow.

As I said earlier, osteoporosis is not a top priority for the NHS, so you may need to take your bone health into your own hands. Ideally, you should book an appointment with a healthcare practitioner (or talk to one on the phone) who can plan a series of tests for you and make recommendations as to what action you should take. He or she can also ensure that, should the tests reveal any underlying problems, you would be referred to an appropriate specialist for further treatment (see page 183 for help in finding a practitioner near you). This could be the only way to ensure that you are not suffering from this 'silent' disease without your knowledge.

Being informed, in my opinion, is the key to good health. If you are tested and find that your bone density is good, this is an indication that you are probably on the right lines in terms of your lifestyle. If, however, you find that your bone density is low, you know that something needs to change if you are to prevent a potential problem from becoming a real one.

Today, people are more proactive than they used to be as far as their health is concerned. Most women want to be better informed about osteoporosis (and their health in general) and the Internet, books and talks all help to make that easier. People are more inclined to ask questions, as opposed to the 'yes sir, no sir' approach of previous generations. It is good to question; if you have even the slightest doubt, or are unsure about anything, you should always ask: What are the benefits of taking this treatment? What are the possible side effects? Are there any risks? What happens if I decide not to take this drug? And, most important of all: What other choices do I have?

Lifestyle changes such as diet, exercise and supplements are all well worth the effort involved and form the cornerstone of a preventative programme for osteoporosis. However, you also need a plan of action for assessing and monitoring your bone health. The steps below will help you to decide what action to take and how to go about it.

STEP 1 – HAVE AN ULTRASOUND BONE SCAN

If you have any of the risk factors listed on page 9, or if you are a woman who is interested in preventing osteoporosis (always a good idea!) or if you just want to know what condition your bones are in, then the first thing you should do is to have a bone scan.

I would recommend an ultrasound bone scan of the heel as a first step. Some ultrasound heel machines are more reliable than others and the better ones reflect more accurately the risk of hip fracture. You may have to organise your scan privately as it is not easy to get one on the NHS (see page 183 for help on where you can get this test). The ultrasound will highlight any bone health problems that may exist, but will also mean that you avoid unnecessary exposure to the X-rays of a DEXA scan, if the results turn out to be normal.

If the scan shows that your bones are:

* normal or osteopenic (low bone density but not osteoporosis), go to Step 3
* osteoporotic, go to Step 2.

STEP 2 – HAVE A DEXA SCAN

As your ultrasound heel bone scan showed signs of osteoporosis, it is important that you have a DEXA scan to look at the density of bone in your hip and spine. A good ultrasound machine will provide an accurate result as the bone at the heel correlates closely with the density at the hip, but you should have this confirmed by having the bones in your spine investigated too.

Your doctor may be able to arrange this scan for you. If you have already had an ultrasound scan that shows signs of osteoporosis and you have other risk factors you might be lucky enough to get a referral for a DEXA scan on the NHS. The length of the waiting list will depend very much on the availability of DEXA scanners in your area. Alternatively, you could arrange for a scan at a private hospital. Cost varies, so shop around. Either way, you should discuss the results with your doctor as you will almost definitely need medical treatment for osteoporosis. It is a good idea to do a bone turnover test before you start on any medication (see Step 3), as this test can monitor the effectiveness of your treatment. At the time of going to press, this test has to be done privately (for further information, see page 32).

Now go to Step 3.

STEP 3 – HAVE A BONE TURNOVER TEST

This test is discussed in more detail on page 32. It cannot diagnose osteoporosis (that is the job of the bone scan which should always be done first), but it does look at the rate of bone loss.

A bone turnover test is a simple non-invasive urine test which measures markers in the urine that are excreted as bone breaks down. The urine sample is collected at home in a kit and then posted to the lab (see page 183 for help on where you can get this test).

If the results of your bone scan show up as either normal or osteopenic your bone turnover results will allow you to see whether or not you are losing bone rapidly on a daily basis.

If your bone turnover is high, action needs to be taken immediately to reduce bone loss and to work on preventing full-blown osteoporosis from developing at any time in the future. Go to Step 4.

If your bone turnover is normal, simply repeat the test every six months to ensure that it stays that way.

If your bone scan shows that you have osteoporosis, then by looking at your bone turnover before you start your medication, you will get a baseline assessment of your bones' rate of resorption before the drug takes effect. If you then repeat the test six weeks after starting your medication, you will be able to see clearly whether or not the drugs are working: quite simply, if your bone turnover is reduced the drugs are working (they are stopping you from losing bone). If your turnover is unchanged, a different medication may be more effective for you.

Even though you are now being medically treated for osteoporosis, you should still go to step 4.

STEP 4 – HAVE A MINERAL ANALYSIS TEST

This simple test, which assesses any deficiencies in the main minerals (calcium, magnesium, zinc), is an incredibly useful tool, whether your bones are normal, osteopenic or osteoporotic (and you are taking medication).

There are many ways of testing for mineral deficiencies, but one of the most helpful ways in terms of bone health is via a hair sample. (A blood sample is not the best medium for testing for calcium deficiency – see page 32.) A high level of calcium in your hair can indicate that calcium is being leached from your bones and dumped in your hair, and a study in 2001 confirmed that abnormal levels of both calcium and phosphorus in hair samples can point to disturbances in bone metabolism.[1]

Hair mineral analysis can assess both deficiencies and excesses in calcium as well as other important minerals such as magnesium, zinc, copper, selenium, chromium, sodium, phosphorus and manganese. It also measures the levels of toxic metals such as mercury, cadmium and aluminium.

Just like any other testing procedure, hair analysis does have its limitations, and certain minerals (iron, for instance) are more accurately tested through a blood sample. But for sufferers of osteoporosis, and those wanting to prevent it, hair analysis remains one of the most relevant – and useful – tests for assessing mineral levels.

Now go to step 5.

STEP 5 – THINK ABOUT YOUR DIGESTIVE SYSTEM

A good, efficient digestive system is crucial in the fight against osteoporosis. It is extremely important that you are able to absorb nutrients from your food and from any supplements you might be taking in order to 'feed' your bones. We know that the production of stomach acid drops as we age, and also that stomach acid plays a vital role in stimulating pancreatic enzymes and releasing bile into the small intestine. These are vital for proper digestion and absorption.

Having any of these symptoms could indicate that a test for digestive function would be useful:

- Do you often feel bloated?
- Do you have a full feeling in your stomach, especially after eating?
- Do you often have wind (flatulence)?
- Do you have irritable bowel symptoms, nervous stomach or loose stools?
- Do you avoid certain foods because they make you feel uncomfortable?
- Are you allergic to any foods?
- Have you ever taken an antibiotic for more than a month at a time or have you taken them more than four times in your life?
- Have you ever taken the Pill, HRT or steroids (cortisone, prednisolone, for example) for extended periods of time?
- Do you have abdominal cramps or pain?
- Do you get heartburn or indigestion or belch after meals?
- Have you ever had food poisoning and found that your bowels have not been 'right' since?

It is important that you check out any symptoms of poor digestion with your doctor. If you are given the all-clear it is worth looking for another approach to solve the problem.

There is a test called a Comprehensive Digestive Stool Analysis (see page 183 for help on where to get this test), which is performed on a stool sample. This would be a particularly useful test if you have any of the risk factors on page 9 and/or a diagnosis of osteoporosis, and if you have answered 'yes' to at least two of the questions above.

The stool analysis reveals:
- how efficiently you are digesting and absorbing food molecules (proteins, fats and starches), with a possible indication of low stomach acid
- whether you have any hidden yeast (candida) and/or bacterial infections
- your levels of friendly, beneficial bacteria in the gut
- the presence of parasites.

Go to Step 6.

STEP 6 – LOOK AT YOUR STRESS LEVELS

As you saw in chapter 5, stress is bad for your bones. Your adrenal glands pump out a number of hormones, one of which is cortisol. Even slightly raised levels of cortisol can increase the risk of fractures, so it is important that stress is controlled as much as possible.

You may not be able to tell how well your body is coping with stress, especially if you go through prolonged stressful periods. If you want to know whether your cortisol levels are too high there is a test that can measure this.

This simple non-invasive test, called an Adrenal Stress Index, is completed by collecting four saliva samples in a kit at home over the course of a day as cortisol is produced at varying levels throughout the day. The samples are then sent back to the lab for analysis. If the test, which can be organised by post (see page 183), shows that your adrenal glands and hormones are out of balance, you will be given recommendations and supplements to help nourish them and get them working appropriately. At the same time you should take steps to see whether you can do anything to control the amount of stress in your life.

Go to Step 7.

STEP 7 – LOOK AT YOUR DIET

There is no doubt that diet plays a critical role in the prevention and treatment of osteoporosis (see chapter 5).

If your bone density is either normal or osteopenic my advice would be to maintain a good healthy diet and put into place as many of the recommendations as you can from chapter 5. The type of diet outlined there will not only help in the prevention of osteoporosis but will also benefit your general health, helping your body to fend off other life-threatening problems such as heart disease and diabetes.

If your bone density is osteoporotic it is even more important for you to follow as many of the recommendations in chapter 5 as you possibly can. Try to switch to, and stay with an alkaline diet on a daily basis. (You can allow yourself the odd indulgence on holiday or at parties – it's what you eat day-today that forms the foundation of your health so a slight lapse here and there should not matter.)

See also chapter 11, Eating for Stronger Bones.

Go to Step 8.

STEP 8 – TAKE FOOD SUPPLEMENTS

Scientific research into vitamins and minerals has been gathering momentum over recent years and we now know exactly which vitamins, minerals and essential fatty acids work best in the fight against osteoporosis (see chapter 6).

If your bone density is normal or osteopenic, I would advise you to take a good programme of supplements (see page 112) to give you enough of the important nutrients to keep your bones healthy and to prevent osteoporosis. Any deficiencies picked up on the mineral analysis test should be supplemented for three months, followed by a retest to check that things are back to normal. Once they are back to normal, you can follow a simple maintenance programme.

If you are osteoporotic, your need for certain vitamins and minerals will be higher and you should follow the recommendations on page 113. Deficiencies picked up on the mineral test should be supplemented at higher levels for three months to get everything back to normal. Once they are back to normal, you only need to stay on a maintenance programme. If your digestion and absorption have been tested and found to be inefficient (see Step 5, above), it is important to take steps to address this; you could be eating a wonderful diet and taking the best supplements in the world, but if your body is not absorbing them it is a wasted effort.

Go to Step 9.

STEP 9 – STEP UP YOUR EXERCISE

Exercise needs to be a priority, not just for your bones but for every aspect of your general health. The benefits of regular exercise cannot be overestimated.

If your bones are normal, focus your exercise routine on prevention. Choose exercises that you enjoy and will keep up on a weekly basis.

If your bones are osteopenic exercise is a bigger priority. You can increase your bone density using a combination of weight-bearing exercise and weight training, as outlined in chapter 7.

If your bones are already osteoporotic exercise is still a priority for you, but you must take care that the exercise you are doing is not causing further damage, and that it is safe for your bones. Walking is great exercise requiring no instruction, but it would be worth seeing a fitness expert who specialises in osteoporosis to find out what other weight-bearing training you can safely do (under instruction). Classes such as Pilates (see page 119) could be very helpful and guidance would be given by the instructor.

PUTTING IT ALL TOGETHER

Osteoporosis is a multifactorial problem and needs to be prevented and treated as such. The best approach is a holistic one, to pull all the different steps mentioned above together.

Conventional medicine often regards us as a group of body parts. There are many different departments in a hospital: rheumatology, ear, nose and throat, gastro-enterology, gynaecological, psychiatric, cardiovascular and so on. But in the human body everything works together and different systems have feedback mechanisms that feed off each other. When one system is thrown out of balance, the others can be and are affected.

For those of you who like to go a step further and have a full check-up, I have designed a special MOT health screening for women (Menopause and Osteoporosis Test) which combines many of the steps above plus much more. After analysis of all the tests you are given a comprehensive, easy-to-read report with an assessment of your state of health around the menopause and your risk of osteoporosis. This includes a detailed, tailor-made, Plan of Action for you to follow, including dietary advice and recommendations for a three-month supplement specifically designed for your individual requirements (see Appendix 4, page 184 for more details).

Genetic tests

There is little point testing for something that you can't do anything about. A good test should give you knowledge, because knowledge is the opportunity for good health. With the advance in the research into genetics, there is now a test that analyses the genetic polymorphisms for osteoporosis that you can modify through diet and lifestyle. This knowledge can reduce the risk of developing osteoporosis and point you towards a treatment that might better suit your genetic make-up (see Chapter 8). This test covers genetic variations that are related to both bone formation and bone resorption and it also covers your genetic tendency towards inflammation because inflammation can increase the risk of osteoporosis.

Where to get the tests

If you are interested in having any of the tests mentioned above you should find a competent healthcare practitioner who can guide you through a structured programme. If you have any difficulties finding someone locally then please feel free to call my clinic where we can check to see if we can recommend anyone near you.

If not, then it is possible for you to do some of these tests by post and we can send you details on how to do this (see page 183 for Clinic contact details).

Chapter 10

Men and Osteoporosis

This book has been written primarily for women because 1 in 3 women over the age of 50 has osteoporosis. Whilst men do get osteoporosis, it only affects 1 man in 9. Having said that, I felt it was important to include a chapter on osteoporosis in men because it does happen, and its causes can be very different from those in women.

The male risk factors for osteoporosis include:

- family history of osteoporosis
- long-term use of corticosteroids
- smoking
- inactivity
- heavy alcohol or caffeine intake
- digestive problems (such as Crohn's, ulcerative colitis or coeliac disease)
- being underweight
- low levels of testosterone
- overactive thyroid.

Some risk factors are common to both men and women, but osteoporosis is less common in men because of differences in the changes in bone density with age. The diagram on page 148 (which also appears on page 17) is important because it shows a number of differences between men and women in terms of bone density.

Both men and women reach their peak bone density at around the age of 25–30. Men, however, are already at an advantage as their bone density is significantly higher than women's at that age, so for them to become osteoporotic they'd have to lose much more bone than women.

Also, as you can see from the diagram, men do not experience the rapid loss of bone around the age of 50 that women do when they hit the menopause. There *is* a decline in bone density for men, but it is much more gradual. It occurs about ten years later than it does in women and it is mirrored by a lowering of sex hormones as they get older. Men lose 15–45 per cent of trabecular bone (the inner, spongy layer of bone, where fractures most commonly occur) over time, compared with 35–50 per cent lost by women.

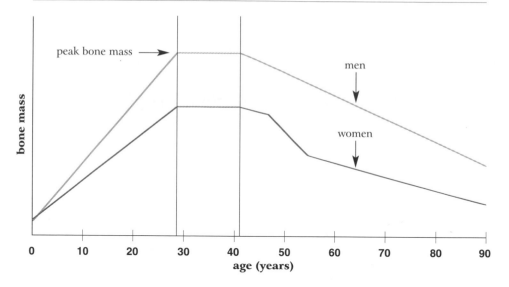

Another factor is that women live longer than men, which gives their bones more time to weaken and increases their lifetime chances of experiencing a fracture.

Although the risk factors listed above for osteoporosis in men do apply, it is thought that in nearly half of the men who get osteoporosis there is no known cause.

In about 20 per cent of men with vertebral fractures the cause is low testosterone. This goes up to 50 per cent in older men with hip fractures.[1] Testosterone triggers the bone-building osteoblasts, and this is accompanied by higher levels of the enzyme, alkaline phosphatase, which helps to form calcium crystals in the bone. As men get older, testosterone levels naturally fall but, in most cases, without the dramatic change in hormones that we see in women at the menopause. For some men, however, testosterone levels become markedly low, causing them to put on weight, feel tired, have reduced sex drive or impotence, and less need to shave.

If a sharp decline in testosterone is suspected, I would recommend a blood test. The sample is usually taken at around 9am as testosterone levels have a circadian rhythm (meaning they follow a 24-hour pattern), rising and falling as the day goes on. They are at their highest in the morning and lowest by 10 in the evening. If the level is below normal it is important to be referred to an endocrinologist so that further tests can be organised to check other hormone levels.

Testosterone can be given as a medication if your levels are naturally low and is taken in the form of tablets, implants or patches. Treatment with testosterone for men with low levels has been shown to increase bone density, by 10 per cent in the spine and 2.7 per cent in the hip.[2] Side effects from testosterone treatment can include acne, decreased HDL ('good' cholesterol) and aggressiveness. The other major concern is the possibility of an increased risk of prostate cancer.

Some scientists have suggested that there might be a male menopause (called an andropause) and that men need testosterone replacement around this time, just as women supposedly 'need' oestrogen. The idea of the andropause is not widely accepted, however, because there is no abrupt change in hormones as there is with *all* women, culminating in a distinct change (that is the end of periods).

SCREENING FOR OSTEOPOROSIS

Testing for osteoporosis is the same for men and women (see chapter 3 for more information). The World Health Organisation's definition of osteoporosis (a T score of below -2.5) is based on post-menopausal women, so strictly speaking it does not apply to men. It has been suggested, however, that there are similarities between bone density and fracture risk in both men and women,[3] so the T score should apply to both and can be used as a guide.

Nowadays, a number of bone scan machines are pre-programmed with bone density data from men, so your T score would then be compared with men at their peak bone density and not post-menopausal women. For real accuracy, I think having the correct comparison is important because otherwise men could always appear to have better bone density than women whose peak bone density is naturally lower.

TREATMENTS FOR OSTEOPOROSIS

It is important to isolate the cause of osteoporosis in men and it is worth seeing a specialist so that a full check-up and blood tests can be performed. If the cause is found to be low testosterone or an overactive thyroid, treatment can be targeted appropriately. If, however, no cause is found, bisphosphonate drugs (see page 42) are routinely prescribed to affected men.

——————— To all women readers ———————

Women who are reading this chapter and who recognise that there is a strong history of osteoporosis in their family for both women and men should tell male family members to be screened for the disease. Many men view osteoporosis as a woman's problem and it is crucial that any risk factors (such as a history of steroid medication) or an inherited link are pointed out to those who should be tested.

THE NUTRITIONAL APPROACH TO OSTEOPOROSIS IN MEN

The chapters in this book on nutrition and supplements are equally applicable to both men and women, so it is really important that those recommendations are put into place. Research into vitamins, minerals and changes in diet has often included both men and women, so the information about an alkaline diet and eating more fruit and vegetables is important for men too.[4] The effects of different foods (like sugar, for example) are also relevant to men[5] and the same goes for supplements like vitamin D and calcium which we know reduce the risk of fractures in men.[6] Furthermore, if these supplements are stopped then the bone density gains are lost over the next 1–2 years (in the case of both men and women).[7]

The same goes for the research on smoking, caffeine and alcohol in that it is applicable to both men and women. The best results are only possible with lifestyle change.

EXERCISE AND OSTEOPOROSIS IN MEN

It was male astronauts who first correlated the gravity-free environment in space with a huge loss in bone density, so clearly the 'use it or lose it' theory applies to men as well as women. Follow the recommendations in chapter 7 and combine both weight-bearing and resistance-training exercises to build bone density.

A good exercise routine is good for your bones, but it is also vital for your heart health. You would certainly stand to lose nothing by putting into place the exercise and other recommendations in this book, and you would have absolutely everything to gain, especially in terms of prevention of further health problems.

Chapter 11

Eating for Stronger Bones

All the different aspects of nutritional advice can become quite confusing, and putting them into practice is a challenge. In this chapter there are guidelines on how to plan bone-restoring meals, and also how to prepare them, using some inspiring osteoporosis-busting recipes. (For more menu-planning ideas, see my cookbook, *Healthy Eating for the Menopause* which includes recipes that are not only helpful as women go through the menopause but are also good for your bones.)

If you are used to a diet consisting largely of highly processed convenience foods, you may well find some of the suggestions here strange at first, but within a few days you will discover just how delicious a wide variety of home-cooked food can really be. You should start feeling healthier and more energised, and within a month or so you will wonder how you ever managed to function on a diet consisting of large amounts of animal protein and refined carbohydrates. Looking after your bones does not have to be all mung beans and broccoli – so read on to find out more.

Most of us do not have much time for preparing meals except, perhaps, when we are expecting guests, so on a day-to-day basis meals need to be quick and easy to prepare, yet still good for your bones. The meals in this chapter are planned on the assumption that you will probably only be cooking for other people in your house once a day and that you are able to choose your own food for breakfast and lunch. Your family do not have to take on your new regime to the same degree but this is generally a healthier way to eat so would be good for them too. You can all eat the same meals but make more dramatic alterations to the acid/alkaline proportions in the food on your own plate. Reduce the size of your portion of animal protein and boost the vegetable part of the meal. Aim to have at least one portion daily of leafy green vegetables (broccoli, cabbage and kale, for example, but not spinach as it blocks calcium absorption), and have either a vegetable/fruit juice or a soup.

Even when you eat out in restaurants you can still emphasise the alkaline part of your diet by ordering extra vegetables and/or a side salad to go with your meal. Choose fish instead of steak or chicken and if you are having an

Indian or Chinese meal, try to have less rice (it will be white rice, and therefore refined) and choose some extra side dishes of vegetables. Both Indian and Chinese restaurants (or takeaways) usually have quite a wide range of vegetable dishes to choose from.

Whilst your main aim should be to make your diet more alkaline, I would also recommend buying organic wherever possible (particularly milk) to ensure that you are getting maximum nutrients from your food without exposing yourself to unnecessary toxins in the form of pesticides or antibiotics.

Have another look at the tables of acid and alkaline foods (see page 62–64) and aim to increase your consumption from the alkaline side little by little each day.

Watch out for the old family favourites, some of which are highly acidic: a meal such as pasta with meat or chicken and cheese sprinkled on the top is a non-starter as cheese is the most acidic of the foods, followed by meat, chicken and pasta. In the PRAL food list, parmesan cheese ranks as the most

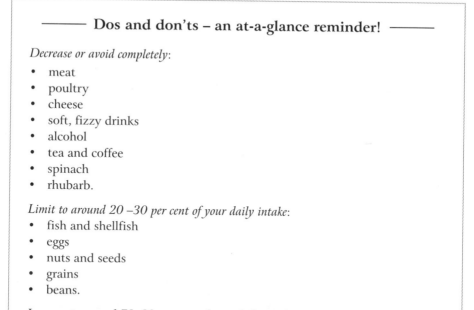

— **Dos and don'ts – an at-a-glance reminder!** —

Decrease or avoid completely:
- meat
- poultry
- cheese
- soft, fizzy drinks
- alcohol
- tea and coffee
- spinach
- rhubarb.

Limit to around 20 –30 per cent of your daily intake:
- fish and shellfish
- eggs
- nuts and seeds
- grains
- beans.

Increase to around 70–80 per cent of your daily intake:
- most fruits and vegetables
- buckwheat
- millet
- sprouted beans/seeds

acidic of all so if you do use it, have only the smallest sprinkling – quantity does make a difference. For an alternative pasta dish, use a good tomato-based pasta sauce (either home-made or an organic sugar-free one from the supermarket or a health-food shop), add salmon (wild or organic, not farmed) to the tomato sauce whilst you cook or heat it and pour this over your pasta. It is delicious served with leafy, green vegetables and a side salad.

My recommendation is to continue eating fish, nuts, grains and beans even though they are in the acid group. You do need *some* acid for your bones, and this way you are choosing healthier sources that also have other benefits for your general health. Whole grains like brown rice are less acidic than white rice because they contain more nutrients as they are not refined. Balance the acidity of those foods by having plenty of fruits and vegetables with them. It is all a question of balance.

The recipes in this chapter put quite a high emphasis on vegetables so that you can increase your vegetable intake without your diet becoming boring. The easiest way to include more vegetables is to have a soup for lunch as often as you can.

Fruit smoothies are a great way of upping your fruit intake. They use whole fruits such as bananas and berries, whizzed in a blender with either orange or apple juice, or you could try organic soya, rice or oat milk or even a live plain organic yoghurt. I always recommend smoothies over fruit or vegetable juices because they contain the whole blended fruit. Juicers extract the juice, and the fibre is discarded. You need fibre, not only to keep things moving through your bowels, but also to help to control blood sugar swings because it slows the passage of food through the digestive system, so preventing a sharp rise in blood sugar. Fibre also helps to reduce cholesterol and is generally beneficial for speeding the removal of waste and harmful toxins.

So whilst juices are fine to drink, they should not be used as a substitute meal. Use them together with other foods so that the juice helps to increase the alkaline balance. A lovely juice that combines vegetables and fruit is a mixture of carrot, apple and raw beetroot. If you can't get raw beetroot, then just use the carrot and apple. You will need a juicer to make these mixes yourself at home – they are better freshly squeezed than bottled – but a bottle of carrot juice (available in most supermarkets and health-food shops) is definitely going to be better than a cola.

Finally, it is important to keep your meals varied. Variety is the key to giving you a good range of vitamins and minerals from food that is both appealing and enjoyable to eat.

BREAKFAST

One of the most acidic breakfasts you could have would be sausages, bacon, eggs, white bread and black coffee with sugar. Many people will just have toast (white) and coffee for breakfast, or even coffee with sugar and a Danish pastry, almond croissant or doughnut (white flour and sugar). None of these options is a good way to start the day. Here are some healthy breakfast suggestions:

Muesli

Choose a good sugar-free muesli and soak it overnight in either apple or orange juice (to break down the phytates in the grains, which stop the absorption of minerals like calcium). Add dried fruit if it is not already in the muesli as this, together with the juice, helps to balance the acidic effect of the grains.

Porridge oats

Cook these with water and top with ground linseeds, or whole or ground sesame or sunflower seeds. You could also add fresh fruit or raisins to increase the alkaline content of the meal, or stir in a teaspoon of sugar-free jam (not diabetic but pure fruit jam available from most supermarkets and health-food shops). Although oats are acid-forming, they are helpful in keeping blood sugar steady and also reducing cholesterol.

Poached/scrambled eggs or a grilled kipper

Serve these with grilled tomatoes and mushrooms which help to offset the acid of the eggs or fish.

Natural live organic yoghurt

Try this with fresh fruit (strawberries or bananas are good), either whipped up into a smoothie or chopped and stirred in. You could also sprinkle some chopped nuts or seeds on the top.

Dried fruit

This should be soaked overnight, and when you buy it choose an organic brand that does not contain sulphur dioxide (this is often added to preserve the colour of apricots, for example, but they taste just as delicious without it). Some dried fruits such as mixed fruit, raisins and sultanas will often have mineral oil added to them to give them a shiny appearance and keep them from sticking together in the bag. Try to avoid this kind of oil as it can interfere with your absorption of calcium and phosphorus which are essential for your bones. As it passes through your body, mineral oil can pick up and excrete the fat-soluble vitamins (A, D, E and K) which your body needs. Buy your dried fruits from either health-food shops or larger supermarkets and check the ingredients carefully.

LUNCH

The most common lunch choice seems to be the humble sandwich. It is not ideal in alkaline terms, but is often the most convenient option, especially when you are eating on the go. Try to balance the acidity of the bread with a fruit snack mid-morning and mid-afternoon.

Some good alkaline fillings for sandwiches would be avocado and salad, hummus and salad, bean sprouts and tahini, tofu mashed with a little miso. Tuna or egg are acceptable as long as you balance them with a decent amount of salad in the sandwich. Try to avoid a white bread sandwich with just ham, beef or chicken. You could always take soup to work with you in a flask, and eat a slice of organic wholewheat or rye bread with it.

A salad is your best possible choice. It's great if you can buy one on the hop, or carry one with you in a container. You could even have hummus, guacamole or lentil pâté (see page 162) with raw vegetable sticks for a perfect lunch. It's easy enough to pick up a tub of hummus from most supermarkets (many now sell organic hummus) and a bag of sliced mixed vegetables (crudités) if you haven't had time to prepare them. Another idea is to take to work a container of leftover food from the previous evening's supper, as long as you have facilities to heat it up thoroughly if required.

When you are at home choosing more alkaline foods is easier. Soups are a great option, particularly vegetable or bean soups. With jacket potatoes, use fillings like tuna, baked beans (you can buy organic tinned baked beans, without sugar, from most supermarkets and health-food shops) or sweet corn (frozen is fine but tinned may contain sugar), and make sure you have a good salad with it.

EVENING MEAL

The aim here is simply to tip the balance of your evening meal so that it becomes more alkaline. An easy way to do this if you are having a piece of grilled fish, for example, is to reduce slightly your fish serving, and give yourself a larger portion of vegetables, both cooked and raw. It is healthier for everyone in the family to reduce the amount of meat in the diet as this has been linked to a higher risk of colon cancer and heart disease.

Introduce small changes gradually, so that you move towards a generally healthier way of eating as a family. Try making a vegetarian dish some evenings, where the protein is coming from the beans, or a risotto accompanied with a side dish of mixed vegetables. Soup can either be a starter to an evening meal or it can be a meal in itself, served with some good-quality bread. Simple stir-fries are quick and easy to make and will give you a good selection of vegetables. Use tamari instead of soya sauce as tamari is wheat-free and helps you to reduce acidity (you can get tamari from health-food shops and some supermarkets also stock it).

Sprouted seeds and beans are useful additions to salads and stir-fries. They are rich in nutrients and easy to digest. You can buy them already grown in packets or grow them yourself. Mung and alfalfa are the easiest to grow: first soak the seeds or beans overnight, then put them in a jar or tray and leave uncovered in a warm, dark place (an airing cupboard is ideal). Rinse the seeds once a day, making sure that all the water is poured off. Before eating, put the seeds in sunlight for several hours, on the window sill and they will turn green. Alternatively, you can buy sprouting kits from most health-food shops.

COOKING TECHNIQUES

Raw vegetables retain the most nutrients but it is good to have a mixture of both raw and cooked. You will find that you need more cooked food when the weather is colder as your body needs the warmth – that is why we tend automatically to go for more salads and raw foods in the summer and soups and stews in the winter. Trying different styles of cooking will help you to include more vegetables in your diet; the way in which you cook your vegetables will alter their taste and make them more interesting.

When cooking vegetables, it is important to try to preserve as much of their goodness as possible, and the best way to achieve this is either to steam them or use a technique called a 'no-water simmer' (below).

No-water simmer

For this method, you need a pan with a tight-fitting lid. Place 2 tablespoons of water in the pan, bring to the boil, then reduce to the lowest possible setting. Add your vegetables, replace the lid and wait 5–10 minutes until all the water has evaporated and the vegetables are cooked. You may need to experiment, to find out exactly how long it takes for your cooker to evaporate 2 tablespoons of water at a low heat.

You can use a wide selection of vegetables and cook them all at the same time. Build layers of vegetables in the pan with onions (finely chopped) first at the bottom, then the more dense vegetables like carrots and parsnips (chopped into smaller pieces so that they cook quicker), followed by cauliflower and/or broccoli and, finally, the leafier vegetables as these will cook the quickest. Add any herbs, garlic or other seasoning that you like – they can be mixed in with the vegetables as you layer them in the pan.

The no-water simmer makes for a fairly 'al dente' type of cooking, but if you prefer your vegetables to be softer, just add a touch more water and leave the lid tightly sealed for longer. It is best to serve the vegetables at once as otherwise they can continue to cook in the heat. Another variation is to add more water and cook the vegetables in layers for about 30 minutes on a low heat in order to bring out their sweetness.

Sautéeing or using a wok

Both these methods require oil. Use olive oil as it is the most stable of the oils and least likely to create free radicals, which have been linked with ageing and cancer. Only fry at low temperatures to reduce the possibility of free radical damage.

Boiling

This is the most wasteful way of cooking vegetables as a lot of valuable nutrients are lost in the cooking water, and it is possibly the least appetising – how many of us still remember our school dinners where the boiled cabbage seemed to be cooked to oblivion. A healthier variation is blanching, where a vegetable is only literally dipped into the boiled water and then removed. My favourite tip is dipping watercress in boiling water. It comes out a bright shade of green and I serve it with lightly roasted sunflower seeds.

Baking

This is a useful method because you can put many different vegetables together in the oven and just leave them whilst you get on with something else. My favourites are baked pumpkin and squash which I either bake whole if there are enough of us to eat it, or slice in half. Potatoes, onions and parsnips can all be baked and baked whole garlic is delicious.

You can also bake fruit: cored eating apples stuffed with raisins and chopped walnuts make an easy dessert.

SOUPS

Soups are really useful as they can often be a meal in themselves, which you can have at lunchtime. They are also a good way of increasing your vegetable intake. The best approach is to cook double the amount that you need and freeze half of it for another time.

Lentil and potato soup

Serves 4

1 tablespoon olive oil
1 large onion, chopped
2 large potatoes, diced
1 dessertspoon tomato purée
850ml (1½ pints) water
60g (2½oz) red lentils
4 large mushrooms, sliced
Bunch of fresh bouquet garni
Soya sauce (tamari) to taste

Stir-fry the onion in the oil until soft, then add the potatoes and fry for a few minutes. Add the tomato purée, then the water and bring to the boil. Add the lentils, mushrooms, herbs and soya sauce to season. Simmer until the potatoes are soft and the lentils cooked. You can either blend this mixture or leave as it is.

Three-bean soup

Serves 4

2 tablespoons olive oil
170g (6oz) onions, chopped
2 cloves garlic, crushed
2 teaspoons ground coriander
1 tablespoon paprika
1 teaspoon mild curry powder
230g (8oz) courgettes, sliced
230g (8oz) potatoes, diced
2 x 400g (14oz) tin of mixed beans (or a packet of mixed beans cooked from
    scratch as instructed on the packet)
1½ litres (2½ pints) water or vegetable stock
340g (12oz) cooked beetroot, diced
Plain yoghurt to serve (optional)

Sauté the onion and garlic in the oil for 2 minutes. Add the spices and cook for another 2 minutes. Add the courgettes and potatoes and cook for a further 2 minutes. Add the drained beans and the water or stock. Cover and simmer for 20 minutes. Add the beetroot, then cook for a further 5 minutes until the potatoes are tender. Blend or serve as it is, depending on preference. Serve on its own or with plain yoghurt.

Other soups

Pumpkin soup and carrot soup are delicious and the method of cooking can be roughly the same:

Sauté onion until soft. Dice the pumpkin or carrots and add to the onions, sautéing for another 5 minutes. Add enough water to cover and simmer until the vegetables are tender. Add more water if needed. The soup can either be eaten as it is or blended to make a smooth soup.

Vegetable soups can also be made with any leftover vegetables. To make a 'cream' soup without using any cream you can use wholemeal flour, cornmeal or any other grain flour to thicken it. Cook a few tablespoons (around 4) of the flour in a little oil for a few minutes until the grain changes colour, then remove the pan from the heat and add in hot stock, or water, and stir quickly. Cook the vegetables separately, then add them to the flour mix. Alternatively, you can cook your vegetables with a small amount of porridge oat flakes which then get blended in with the vegetables and thicken the soup.

VEGETABLE AND BEAN DISHES

Oriental vegetables

Serves 4

170g (6oz) creamed coconut
$^1/_2$ teaspoon salt
600ml (1 pint) hot water
2 tablespoons olive oil
170g (6oz) shiitake mushrooms
1cm ($^1/_2$in) root ginger, finely chopped
3 cloves garlic, finely chopped
2 fresh red chillies (optional), deseeded and thinly sliced
300g (10$^1/_2$oz) cherry tomatoes, halved
115g (4oz) baby sweetcorn, cut in half lengthways
250g (9oz) tin of water chestnuts, drained and sliced
1 bunch of spring onions, thinly sliced
250g (9oz) bean sprouts
1 cos lettuce, sliced thinly into 2.5cm (1in) strips
8 tablespoons lemon juice
Handful of fresh mint, chopped
Handful of fresh coriander, chopped

Place the creamed coconut and salt into a measuring jug, add the hot water and stir until the coconut has dissolved.

Heat the oil in a wok. Add the mushrooms and stir for 1–2 minutes until they start to soften. Stir in the ginger and garlic, then the chillies. Add the cherry tomatoes, baby sweetcorn and water chestnuts and then pour in the coconut milk.

Bring the mixture to the boil and leave bubbling for 2 minutes, then add the spring onions and bean sprouts. Add the lettuce and stir until just wilted. Stir in the lemon juice and then the chopped herbs. Serve immediately with brown rice.

Cucumber dill salad

4 tablespoons tahini (sesame seed paste)
125ml (4fl oz) water
5 teaspoons lemon juice
2 teaspoon soya sauce or tamari
Several pinches of dry dill or $^1/_2$ teaspoon of fresh chopped dill
570g (1$^1/_4$lb) cucumber, peeled, scored (run a fork along the side) and sliced

Mix the tahini and water until smooth. Add the lemon, tamari and dill. Mix the cucumber slices with the other ingredients. This dish can taste even better the next day as it will have marinated overnight.

Tofu bake

Serves 4

170g (6oz) tofu, diced
1 tablespoon soya sauce or tamari
750g (1lb 10oz) potatoes, chopped
2 tablespoons olive oil
230g (8oz) leeks, chopped
1 garlic clove, crushed
1 large aubergine, diced
170g (6oz) mushrooms, chopped
1 teaspoon thyme
1 teaspoon oregano
1 tablespoon wholemeal flour
300ml (½ pint) water or vegetable stock
1 tablespoon sesame seeds

Marinate the tofu by pouring the soya sauce over it and leave to stand for
30 minutes. Bring enough water to the boil to cover the potatoes and cook
until soft. Mash them and leave to one side.

Heat the oil in a frying pan and add the leeks, garlic and aubergine and
cook until tender. Add the mushrooms, thyme and oregano and cook for a
further 2–3 minutes. Sprinkle the flour over the vegetables, stir over the heat
and cook for 1–2 minutes. Gradually add the water or stock, bring to the boil
and add the tofu and soya sauce. Simmer for 5 minutes.

Pour the vegetable mixture into the bottom of an ovenproof dish, spread
the potatoes over the top, sprinkle on the sesame seeds and bake for
30 minutes in a preheated oven at 190°C/375°F/gas 5.

Sweet and sour red cabbage

Serves 4

1 litre (1¾ pints) water
2 onions, sliced
4 apples, sliced
6 tablespoons sultanas
2 red cabbages, finely shredded

In a heavy pan, bring the water to the boil, add the onions and cook for
2 minutes. Add the apples, sultanas and red cabbage. Cover and cook until
tender, about 30 minutes.

Guacamole

1 small onion
1 x 150g (5oz) carton natural organic live yoghurt
1 large, ripe avocado, peeled and stoned
1 tablespoon lemon juice
Freshly ground pepper
2 tomatoes, chopped

Place the onion in a food processor and process until finely chopped. Add the yoghurt, avocado, lemon juice and pepper. Process until smooth. Add the chopped tomatoes and process until blended.

Red lentil pâté

145g (5oz) red lentils
700ml (1¼ pints) water
2 tablespoons olive oil
115g (4oz) onion, diced
2 garlic cloves, crushed
½ teaspoon dried marjoram
1 tablespoon lemon juice
3 tablespoons fresh parsley, chopped
1 tablespoon fresh basil, chopped
2 teaspoons miso, thinned in 2 teaspoons water

Wash and drain the lentils. Bring to the boil with the water, then simmer, covered, for about 30 minutes, until tender. Simmer for a further 10 minutes or until nearly all the liquid has been absorbed.

Heat 1 tablespoon of the oil and sauté the onion and garlic until soft. Add the marjoram and sauté for 1 minute. Add this mixture to the lentils, then add the remaining ingredients and blend until mixed well.

Allow to cool before serving; the pâté will thicken as it cools and will last for almost a week in the fridge. Brilliant for lunch!

Guacamole and hummus are good lunch-time stand-bys to eat with raw vegetables.

You can buy organic hummus or make your own – there is a lovely humous recipe in my *Healthy Eating for the Menopause* cookbook.

SALADS

Vegetable salad
2 carrots, cut into matchsticks
2 celery sticks, cut into matchsticks
1 red, 1 yellow, 1 orange and 1 green pepper, all sliced thinly
1 teaspoon maple syrup
1 tablespoon fresh mint, chopped

Dressing
1 teaspoon fresh mint, chopped
2 tablespoons walnut oil
1 tablespoon cider vinegar
1 teaspoon wholegrain mustard

Mix together all the salad ingredients. Whisk together the salad dressing
ingredients. Toss the salad with the dressing.

Sprouted salad
Packet of mixed sprouted seeds or beans
1 red pepper, sliced
1 green pepper, sliced

Mix together salad ingredients and stir in French dressing (below).

French dressing
Juice of 1 lemon
50ml (2fl oz) cider vinegar
225ml (8fl oz) olive oil

Whisk all the ingredients together.

Alfalfa sprout salad

Banana
Lemon juice
Alfalfa sprouts
Walnuts
Raisins
Sliced apples

There are no quantities for this recipe, so the aim is to use the ingredients and
alter the balance to get the taste you prefer. Mash a banana and add lemon
juice to make the consistency thinner. Add to the alfalfa sprouts and also add
walnuts, raisins and sliced apples to get a lovely mixture.

GRAIN DISHES

Millet

This is an alkaline grain, so it is very useful and very light.

Basic millet

145g (5oz) millet, washed and drained
480ml (16fl oz) water
pinch of sea salt

Dry roast the millet in a pan until it is fragrant and starts to pop (about 10 minutes). Add the water and salt and bring to the boil. Lower the heat, cover and simmer for 40 minutes. Fluff with a fork before serving.

Millet and cauliflower mash

Serves 4

water
2 tablespoons soya sauce or tamari
2 medium cauliflowers, cut into florets
1.5 litres (2½ pints) water
290g (10oz) millet

To a heated pan, add the oil and onions and stir until tender. Add the soya sauce and stir again. Add the cauliflower, water and millet. Bring to a boil and cook on a low flame for 30 minutes. When cooked, mash the mixture and serve with leafy green vegetables.

Grilled millet rissoles

Serves 4

145g (5oz) millet
700ml (1¼ pints) water
1 medium sweet potato, chopped
1 teaspoon mustard seeds
1 teaspoon curry powder
1 teaspoon fresh ginger, grated
½ cup fresh coriander, chopped

Toast the millet in a heavy pan until it starts to smell fragrant. Leave aside. Put the water, sweet potato, mustard seeds, curry and ginger into a saucepan and bring to the boil. Add the toasted millet. Cover and reduce heat and cook for 25–30 minutes or until the millet has absorbed all the water. Allow to cool.

With your hands, mix the coriander into the millet. Form into small rissoles and grill under a medium heat, until each side is golden. Can be served with a salad and/or a green vegetable such as broccoli.

Brown rice

Brown rice provides more nutrients than white because it is a wholefood. Use it in recipes where you would previously have used white rice. It is usual to have long-grain brown rice in summer and the heartier short grain in the winter. Just allow a little more time for preparing your meal as brown rice takes longer than white to cook.

I always cook more brown rice than I need for a meal because leftover rice, once cool, will keep for several days in the fridge and can be used for quick lunches or dinner. To heat up leftover rice, either sauté in a little oil and add tamari, or steam the rice in a small-holed vegetable steamer over boiling water until thoroughly reheated.

Curried rice

Serves 4

1 tablespoon olive oil
1 onion, chopped
1 teaspoon mild curry powder
60g (2oz) raisins
60g (2oz) blanched almonds, finely chopped
230g (8oz) cooked brown rice

Heat the oil in a frying pan and fry the onion for 5 minutes until soft. Add the curry powder and cook, stirring for 1 minute. Add the raisins and almonds and stir well. Add the rice and combine well. Cook over a low heat, stirring for 1–2 minutes or until the rice is heated through.

Quinoa

Quinoa contains high levels of minerals and is a good source of vegetable protein, quick and easy to prepare. It is used as an accompaniment instead of rice or pasta. It can also be used in desserts, such as an alternative to rice pudding (see below).

Basic preparation of quinoa

Serves 4

480ml (16fl oz) water
Tiny pinch of sea salt
145g (5oz) quinoa

Always use twice as much water as quinoa. Place the water and salt in a pan and bring to the boil. Add the quinoa, cover, reduce to a simmer and cook for 15–20 minutes or until the water is absorbed. Remove from the heat. Allow to rest, covered, for 5–10 minutes and then fluff with a fork.

Quinoa pudding

Serves 4

480ml (16fl oz) water
145g (5oz) quinoa, rinsed
2 tablespoons tahini
2 tablespoons maple syrup
2 eggs, lightly beaten
480ml (16fl oz) soya milk
1 tablespoons vanilla
$1/4$ tablespoon grated lemon zest
45g ($1\frac{1}{2}$ oz) dates, chopped
45g ($1\frac{1}{2}$ oz) currants
45g ($1\frac{1}{2}$ oz) toasted ground almonds
Freshly grated nutmeg

Bring the water to the boil and add the quinoa. Lower heat and cook for 10 minutes or until the water is absorbed. Allow to sit for 5 minutes. Preheat oven to 160°C/325°F/gas 3. Cream the tahini with the maple syrup. Stir in the eggs, soya milk, vanilla and lemon zest. Add quinoa, then the dates and currants and mix well. Oil a casserole dish and sprinkle the bottom with 2 tablespoons of the nuts. Pour in quinoa mixture and top with the remaining nuts and nutmeg. Bake for 50 minutes or until set.

FISH DISHES

Roasted cod

Serves 4

4 cod fillets (150g/5½ oz) each
8 tablespoons olive oil
2 tablespoons cumin
2 teaspoons turmeric
1 onion, chopped
1 garlic clove, crushed
2 potatoes, diced
2 carrots, diced
125g (4½oz) pumpkin, diced
1 teaspoon ground ginger
1 teaspoon cinnamon
400g (14oz) tin of cannellini beans, drained
50g (2oz) pre-soaked prunes
120ml (4fl oz) water

Marinate the cod with 4 tablespoons olive oil, the cumin and turmeric and refrigerate for 1 hour (if time is short then just brush the cod with olive oil before roasting).

Heat the remaining oil in a frying pan, add the onion and garlic and sweat until tender. Add the potatoes, carrots and pumpkin and fry until golden. Add the ginger and cinnamon, reduce the heat and cook gently for 5 minutes. Add the beans, prunes and water and cook until all the vegetables are tender.

Place the fish in a roasting tin, brush with the marinade or just olive oil (if you haven't had time to marinate it) and roast for 5–8 minutes at 200°C/400°F/gas 6. Serve with the vegetables.

Fish stew

Serves 8

1 medium onion, diced
1 carrot, diced
1 stick of celery, sliced
1.5 litres (2½ pints) water
455g (1lb) cod or salmon
1 tablespoon fresh ginger, grated
2 tablespoons tamari or soya sauce

Put the onion, carrot and celery in a heavy saucepan with the water and simmer for 20 minutes, stirring often.

Cut the cod into large pieces and add to the pot together with the ginger and tamari. Cover and simmer for a further 10–15 minutes.

You can ring the changes with this dish by adding different vegetables. To vary the taste you can also sauté the onions first with oil in the bottom of the pan and then add the other vegetables and water and continue as before.

FRUIT DISHES

Fruit jelly

Jellies are usually made from gelatine which comes from the boiled down hooves of cattle. They may also contain colouring and sugar or artificial sweeteners so it is good to have alternatives. Fruit jelly made with real fruit juice is wonderful on a summer's day (for adults as well as children) and can be used to accompany a fruit salad.

For a colourful jelly use red grape juice or diluted blackcurrant (make sure that the juice you buy does not contain sugar or colourings). Bring 300ml ($^1/_2$ pint) of juice to the boil and add 1 teaspoon of agar powder (this is a form of seaweed which you can buy in health-food shops). Once the agar has dissolved, transfer to a dish or mould. It can be left to set at room temperature and as it sets you can add halves of seedless grapes or berries.

Nectarines with raspberries

8 tablespoons orange juice
3 tablespoons maple syrup (the real stuff, not maple flavoured)
4 nectarines, thinly sliced
145g (5oz) chilled raspberries
2 tablespoons sliced almonds, toasted

Bring the orange juice and maple syrup to the boil in a heavy pan. Add the nectarines and cook, turning occasionally, for about 5 minutes until the fruits soften. Use a slotted spoon to transfer the nectarines to a bowl. Simmer the juice left in the pan until it thickens, about 2 minutes. Pour the thickened juice over the nectarines and leave to cool for at least 10 minutes. When ready to serve, stir the raspberries in with the warm nectarines. Serve in individual bowls, with a sprinkling of toasted almonds.

Stewed fruit

You can make a lovely hot fruit dessert simply by mixing chopped eating apples and raisins and cooking them up together.

For a more adventurous version, use apples or pears, dates and raisins and simmer slowly for about 15 minutes. Cinnamon or other spices can be added to fruit whilst it is cooking. Lemon and walnuts added to the mixture also make a nice variation.

Apple crumble

Serves 8

For the topping:
1 ¹/₂ teaspoon cinnamon
¹/₂ teaspoon nutmeg
3 tablespoons cold-pressed unrefined corn oil
3 tablespoons maple syrup
200g (7oz) whole wheat flour

For the filling:
1 tablespoon corn oil
800g (1 ³/₄ lb) apples, thinly sliced (use eating rather than cooking apples so that they won't need sweetening)
45g (1 ¹/₂ oz) raisins
4 tablespoons lemon or apple juice
4 tablespoons maple syrup (once you have tried this you may find that it is sweet enough without the maple syrup)
1 tablespoon vanilla essence

Preheat oven to 180°C/350°F/gas 4. Mix all the topping ingredients apart from the flour, then add to the flour. Stir, then rub the mixture between your palms until it is crumbly. Spread on a baking sheet and bake until the mixture dries out a bit, about 10 minutes.

To make the filling, heat the oil and sauté the apples briefly to coat. Add the other ingredients, stir and cook over medium heat, uncovered, until the apples soften, about 10 minutes, stirring occasionally.

Oil an 20cm (8in) square baking dish with corn oil, add the filling, spread over the topping and bake for 20 minutes.

─────────── Shopping list for alkaline foods ───────────

Vegetables

Aubergines, beetroots, broccoli, Brussels sprouts, cabbage, carrots, cauliflower, celery, cucumbers, garlic, kale, lettuce, mushrooms, onions, parsnips, peppers, potatoes, pumpkin, seaweeds, spring greens, squash, sweet potatoes, watercress.

Fruit

Apples, apricots, avocados, bananas, blackberries, blueberries, cherries, currants, dates, figs, grapefruit, grapes, lemons, limes, loganberries, mangoes, melon, nectarines, olives, oranges, papayas, peaches, pears, pineapples, raisins, raspberries, strawberries, tangerines, tomatoes, watermelon.

Grains

Buckwheat, millet.

Nuts

Almonds, Brazil nuts.

Dairy

Organic yoghurt, milk.

Drinks

Fruit and vegetable juice, green tea, herb and fruit teas, Rooisbosch (red bush) tea, water.

Note: vegetable oils and butter are neutral.

Remember to choose brown rice, porridge oats and other whole grains as the less refined the grain, the more alkaline it becomes. Also include nuts, seeds and legumes as these are good for your general health and are also good-quality acid ash foods (see page 62) as you do need some acid foods in your diet.

Table of PRAL values of different foods (for 100g of each food)[1]

Food Groups	Highly Acid	Acid	Alkaline	Highly Alkaline
Vegetables			Asparagus -0.4	Spinach -14.0
			Aubergine -3.4	
			Broccoli (green) -1.2	
			Carrots -4.9	
			Cauliflower -4.0	
			Celery -5.2	
			Chicory -2.0	
			Courgettes -4.6	
			Cucumber -0.8	
			Leeks -1.8	
			Lettuce (average of 4 varieties) -2.5	
			Lettuce (iceberg) -1.6	
			Mushroom (common) -1.4	
			Onions -1.5	
			Peppers (*Capsicum*, green) -1.4	
			Potatoes -4.0	
			Radish (red) -3.7	
			Tomato Juice -2.8	
			Tomatoes -3.1	

Food Groups	Highly Acid	Acid	Alkaline	Highly Alkaline
Fruits and Fruit Juices			Apple juice (unsweetened) -2.2	Raisins -21.0
			Apples (15 varieties, flesh and skin, average) -2.2	
			Apricots -4.8	
			Bananas -5.5	
			Blackcurrants -6.5	
			Cherries -3.6	
			Grape Juice (unsweetened) -1.0	
			Kiwi fruit -4.1	
			Lemon juice -2.5	
			Orange juice (unsweetened) -2.9	
			Oranges -2.7	
			Peaches -2.4	
			Pears (3 varieties, flesh and skin, average) -2.9	
			Pineapple -2.7	
			Strawberries -2.2	
			Watermelon -1.9	

Food Groups	Highly Acid	Acid	Alkaline	Highly Alkaline
Grain Products		Bread (rye flour, mixed) 4.0		
		Bread (rye flour) 4.1		
		Bread (wheat flour, mixed) 3.8		
		Bread (wheat flour, wholemeal) 1.8		
		Bread (white wheat) 3.7		
		Cornflakes 6.0		
		Crispbread (rye) 3.3		
		Noodles (egg) 6.4		
		Oats 10.7		
		Rice (brown) 12.5		
		Rice (white, easy cook) 4.6		
		Rice (white, easy cook, boiled) 1.7		
		Rye flour (whole) 5.9		
		Spaghetti (white) 6.5		
		Spaghetti (whole meal) 7.3		
		Wheat flour (white, plain) 6.9		
		White flour (whole meal) 8.2		

Food Groups	Highly Acid	Acid	Alkaline	Highly Alkaline
Dairy Products		Buttermilk 0.5 Camembert 14.6		
	Cheddar cheese 26.4			
		Cheese (Gouda) 18.6		
		Cottage cheese 8.7		
		Creams (fresh, sour) 1.2		
		Fresh cheese 11.1		
		Full-fat soft cheese 4.3		
	Hard cheese (average of 4 types) 19.2			
		Ice cream (dairy, vanilla) 0.6		
		Milk (whole, evaporated) 1.1		
		Milk (whole, pasteurised and sterilised) 0.7		
	Parmesan 34.2			
	Processed cheese (plain) 28.7			
		Yoghurt (whole milk, fruit) 1.2		
		Yoghurt (whole milk, plain) 1.5		

Food Groups	Highly Acid	Acid	Alkaline	Highly Alkaline
Animal Products	Eggs (yolk) 23.4	Beef 7.8		
		Chicken 8.7		
		Cod 7.1		
		Corned beef (tinned) 13.2		
		Eggs (chicken, whole) 8.2		
		Eggs (white) 1.1		
		Frankfurters 6.7		
		Haddock 6.8		
		Herring 7.0		
		Liver sausage 10.6		
		Luncheon meat (tinned) 10.2		
		Pork 7.9		
		Rump steak (lean and fat) 8.8		
		Salami 11.6		
		Trout 10.8		
		Turkey 9.9		
		Veal (fillet) 9.0		
Legumes			Green beans -3.1	
		Lentils 3.5		
		Peas 1.2		
			Soya beans -4.7	

Food Groups	Highly Acid	Acid	Alkaline	Highly Alkaline
Nuts			Hazelnuts -2.8	
		Peanuts 8.3		
		Walnuts 6.8		
Drinks			Beer (draught) -0.2	
		Beer (pale) 0.9		
			Beer (stout, bottled) -0.1	
		Cola 0.4		
			Cocoa (made with semi-skimmed milk) -0.4	
			Coffee -1.4	
			Mineral water (Apollinaris) -1.8	
			Mineral water (Volvic) -0.1	
			Red wine -2.4	
			Tea -0.3	
			White wine -1.2	

Food Groups	Highly Acid	Acid	Alkaline	Highly Alkaline
Other Foods		Butter 0.6		
		Chocolates (milk) 2.4		
			Honey -0.3	
			Margarine -0.5	
		Madeira cake 3.7		
			Marmalade -1.5	
			Olive oil neutral at 0.0	
			Sugar (white) -0.1	
			Sunflower seed oil neutral at 0.0	

Appendix 1

Glossary

Acid/alkaline ash – the residue left by the mineral content of food which can be used to determine that food's acidity/alkalinity

Acidosis – name given to state in which blood pH falls below 7.35

Alkalosis – name given to state in which blood pH rises above 7.45

Amino acids – 25 nitrogen-bearing molecules that form the basis of proteins, eight of which are known as 'essential'

Antioxidant – a substance occurring naturally in the food you eat which protects against the harmful effects of free radicals

Biochemical markers – microscopic 'clues' in the blood and urine that can show the rate of bone turnover

Bisphosphonates – these are widely used as non-hormonal 'anti-resorptive' drugs in the treatment of osteoporosis

Bone loss – this occurs when the rate of bone renewal does not keep up with the rate of its breakdown

Bone matrix – the architecture of the bone

Bone resorption – the process by which old or damaged bone is dissolved

Bone turnover – the rate at which bone is dissolved and renewed

Bone turnover analysis – tests on blood or urine that monitor bone loss and can be used in the diagnosis and treatment of osteoporosis

Calcitonin – a natural hormone produced by the thyroid gland; it inhibits the cells which break down bone

Calcitriol – a naturally occurring active form of vitamin D (also available in synthetic form); vitamin D is essential for calcium absorption

CAT scan – a scanner used to measure bone density

Coeliac disease – a digestive disorder characterised by gluten intolerance

Collagen – a major bone protein that acts as a 'cement', holding the bone matrix together

Cortical bone – the dense, outer layer of bone

Cytokine – powerful 'signal' molecule which transfer information from one cell or organ to another

DNA (deoxyribonucleic acid) – molecules that carry genetic information and control the inheritance of characteristics

DEXA scan (Dual Energy X-ray Absorptiometry) – a machine that uses two X-ray energy beams (one high- and one low-energy) simultaneously

Free radicals – chemically unstable atoms that can cause damage in your body; pollution, smoking, fried or barbecued food and UV rays from the sun can all trigger free radicals

Genomics – the study of genes and their function

Genotype – a person's genetic make-up

Homocysteine – a toxic by-product of the breakdown of one of the amino acids (methionine)

HRT – hormone replacement therapy

Kyphosis – an outward curving of the spine (also known as a dowager's hump), causing loss of height

Oestrogen – female hormone secreted by the ovaries

Oestrone – a weak form of oestrogen

Osteoblasts – bone-building cells; their job is to fill the cavities left by the removal of old bone

Osteocalcin – a bone-building protein

Osteoclasts – cells which break down bone; they work to dissolve slowly old or damaged bone

Osteopenia – the stage at which your bones are below normal but not yet osteoporotic

Osteoporosis – literally 'porous bones'; a disease occurring when, over a period of years, the rate of bone renewal does not keep up with the rate of its breakdown, resulting in bones that are filled with tiny pores or holes

Peak bone density – the point at which you have as much bone as you will ever have (occurs around the age of 25); the higher your peak bone density, the lower your risk of osteoporosis in later life

pH (potential Hydrogen) – a measure of a solution's acidity/alkalinity

Phenotype – the individual identifying traits of a person, such as their height, blood group or sex

Phytoestrogens – substances which occur naturally in food and which have a weak oestrogenic activity, allowing them to behave in a similar way to SERMs (see below)

Polymorphism – a small variation in the genetic code that can be passed down through generations

PRAL (Potential Renal Acid Load) – a calculation used to measure the acid/alkaline effects of food on the kidneys

Progesterone – a hormone naturally produced by the ovaries

SERMS (Selective Oestrogen Receptor Modulators) – new, designer HRTs intended to provide the beneficial effects of oestrogen where needed (i.e. the bones), whilst avoiding any stimulating effects in areas where too much oestrogen can be dangerous (e.g. the breasts and womb)

SNP (single-nucleotide polymorphism) – a change in the DNA sequence that involves a variation in a single nucleotide (one of the structural building blocks of DNA)

Soya isolates – isolated compounds of soya which bear little similarity to the original soya bean

T score – the difference between your bone density and that of the average 25-year-old woman at peak bone density; in other words how far off the ideal you are

Teriparatide – a new drug used to activate bone-building in the treatment of osteoporosis

Testosterone – a hormone produced by the ovaries

Trabecular bone – the inner 'spongy' layer of bone

Ultrasound scan – also known as QUS or quantitative ultrasound scan, this passes sound waves through the heel bone to measure factors such as bone stiffness/elasticity

Z score – your bone density compared with that of other women of the same age as you; this is 'age-matched', in other words how you compare with your peers

Appendix 2

Useful Addresses

Acupuncture
The British Acupuncture Council
63 Jeddo Road
London W12 9HQ
Tel: 020 8735 0400

Homeopathy
Society of Homeopaths
4a Artizan Road
Northampton NN1 4HU
Tel: 01604 621400

Medical Herbalism
National Institute of Medical
Herbalism
56 Longbrook Street
Exeter EX4 6AH
Tel: 01392 42602

Nutrition
British Association for Nutritional
Therapy
27 Old Gloucester Street
London WC1N 3XX
Tel: 0870 6061284

Osteopathy
General Osteopathic Council
Osteopathy House
176 Tower Bridge Road
London SE1 3LU
Tel: 020 7357 6655

Osteoporosis
National Osteoporosis Society
Camerton
Bath BA2 OPJ
Tel: 01761 471771

Premature Menopause
The Daisy Network
PO Box 392
High Wycombe
Bucks HP15 7SH

Yoga
The British Wheel of Yoga
1 Hamilton Place
Boston Road
Sleaford
Lincs NG34 7ES
Tel: 01529 306851

Alexander Technique
The Society of Teachers of the
Alexander Technique
20 London House
266 Fulham Road
London SW10 9EL
Tel: 020 7351 0828

Pilates
The Body Control Pilates Association
6 Langley Street
London WC2H 9JA
Tel: 020 7379 3734

Appendix 3

The Dr Marilyn Glenville Clinic
Natural healthcare for women

If you would like more information or would like to see a practitioner regarding the natural approach to osteoporosis including:

- Bone scans
- Menopause and Osteoporosis Test (MOT)
- Genetic testing
- Mineral analysis
- Digestive stool analysis

and any other tests mentioned in this book, then please feel free to phone my clinic.

Consultations
Private and telephone consultations are available at my **London** or **Tunbridge Wells** clinics. For appointments and enquiries please contact:

The Dr Marilyn Glenville Clinic
14 St Johns Road
Tunbridge Wells
Kent TN4 9NP

Tel: 0870 5329244 / Fax: 0870 5329255
International: Tel: +44 1 892 515905 / **Fax:** + 44 1 892 515914

Email: health@marilynglenville.com
Website: www.marilynglenville.com

MOT Health Screen
(Menopause and Osteoporosis Test)

This is an exclusive range of tests that I have put together to help you find out your current state of health around the menopause.

Here's the range of tests the MOT health screen includes:

- Bone ultrasound scan
- Bone turnover test
- Mineral test
- Cholesterol test – including HDL, LDL and triglycerides
- Diabetes test
- Blood pressure measurement
- Height and weight assessment
- Body fat assessment
- BMI index
- Homocysteine measurement
- Oestrogen metabolism test
- Consultation with a qualified practitioner
- Full written report with results of all your tests, specific dietary recommendations and recommendations for a tailor-made three-month supplement programme.

You can have the full MOT package which includes all the tests above or pick and choose the tests you want depending on your circumstances.

How is the MOT screening different from other screens?

The MOT screening is different from the usual Well Woman screen, conducted by your doctor or medical insurance company because it is aimed at women around the time of the menopause who are interested in picking up potential problems and who are committed to prevention. It checks for nutritional deficiencies that are not included on a Well Woman screen and measures other markers such as bone turnover and homocysteine that are invaluable for highlighting future osteoporosis, heart and other problems.

Detailed dietary recommendations are given together with recommendations for a three-month programme of supplements to correct any deficiencies and to focus on any other problems that may be picked up. You will be given a full report with all copies of your test results and all the recommendations given are summarised in a tailor-made Plan of Action for you so you can refer to them any time to help keep you on track.

If you are interested in having an MOT health screen, then please call my clinic for more information (see page 183 for clinic contact details).

Appendix 5

Genetic Testing

The particular predictive genetics test I recommend for osteoporosis measures a range of polymorphisms relating to bone health and osteoporosis risk. The polymorphisms it measures are:

- Collagen type 1 alpha 1 (COL1A1)
- Calcitonin receptor (CALCR)
- Vitamin D3 receptor (VDR)
- Interleukin-6 (IL-6)
- Tumour necrosis factor-alpha (TNF-alpha)

A kit is sent to you and your cells are collected using either a mouth rinse or by a blood sample which you then send directly to the laboratory. Your results are then sent back to your practitioner. Because these are genetic tests, the results must always be discussed face to face in the clinic. This cannot be done on the telephone.

If you are interested in finding out what your genetic profile suggests is the best treatment for you, then please call my clinic for more information (see page 183 for clinic contact details).

References

Introduction

1   Gallagher, T.C. *et al.*, 2002, 'Missed opportunities for prevention of osteoporotic fracture', *Arch Intern Med*, 162, 45–456.
2   Wilson, J.M.G. and Junger, G., 1968, *Principles and practice of screening for disease*, World Health Organisation, Geneva.
3   Mazanec, D., 2004, 'Osteoporosis screening – time to take responsibility', *Arch Int Med*, 1047–48.

Chapter 1

1   Jonsson, B. *et al.,* 1999, 'Effect and offset of treatments for hip fracture on health outcomes', *Osteoporosis International*, 10, 193-9.
2   Gourlay, M.L. and Brown, S.A., 2004, 'Clinical considerations in premenopausal osteoporosis', *Arch Intern Med*, 164, 603–14.
3   Gail, A. *et al.,* 2000, 'How many women lose bone mineral density while taking hormone replacement therapy?' Results from the Postmenopausal Estrogen/Progestin Interventions Trial, *Archives of Internal Medicine*, 160, 3065–71.
4   Gilsanz, V. *et al.*, 1991, 'Changes in vertebral bone density in black girls and white girls during childhood and puberty', *New England Journal of Medicine*, 325, 1597–1600.
5   Martin, M.C. *et al.*, 1993, 'Menopause without symptoms: The endocrinology of menopause among rural Mayan Indians', *American Journal of Obstetrics and Gynaecology*, 168, 6, 1839–45.
6   Lees, B. *et al.,* 1993, 'Differences in proximal femur bone density over two centuries', *Lancet*, 341, 8846, 673–5.

Chapter 2

1   McGuigan, F.E.A. *et al.*, 2001, 'Prediction of osteoporotic fractures by bone densitometry and COL1A1 genotyping: a prospective, population-based study in men and women', *Osteoporosis Int*, 12, 91–6.
2   Health and Welfare Canada, 1993, Canada's Health Promotion Survey 1990: Technical Report, Minister of Supply and Services, Ottawa.
3   Schreiber, G.B. *et al.*, 1996, 'Weight medication effects reported by black and white preadolescent girls, National Heart, Lung and Blood Institute Growth and Health Study, *Paediatrics*, 98, 1, 63–70.
4   Kann, L. *et al.*, 1998, 'Youth risk behaviour surveillance – United States, 1997', *Morb. Mortal. Weekly Rep.*, 47 (SS-3), 1–89.
5   Lennkh, C. *et al.*, 1999, 'Osteopenia in anorexia nervosa: specific mechanisms of bone loss', *J. Psychiatr. Res.*, 33, 349–56.

6   KinK, *et al.*, 1991, 'Bone mineral density of the spine in normal Japanese subject using DEXA: effect of obesity and menopausal status', *Calcification Tissue International*, 49, 101–6.

7   Law, M.R. and Hackshaw, A.K., 1997, 'A meta-analysis of cigarette smoking, bone mineral density and risk of hip fracture: recognition of a major effect', *British Medical Journal*, 315, 841–6.

8   Di Prospero, F. *et al.*, 2004, 'Cigarette smoking damages women's reproductive life', *Reprod Biomed Online*, 8, 2, 246–7.

9   Francis, R., 1998, 'Management of corticosteroid-induced osteoporosis', *Journal of the British Menopause Society*, 4, 2, 52–6.

10   2002, *Glucocorticoid Induced Osteoporosis: Guidelines for Prevention and Treatment*, Royal College of Physicians, London.

11   Israel, E. *et al.*, 2001, 'Effects of inhaled glucorticoids on bone density in premenopausal women', *New England Journal of Medicine*, 2001, 345, 941–7.

12   Fujita, K., 2001, 'Inhaled corticosteroids reduce bone mineral density in early postmenopausal but premenopausal asthmatic women', *J. Bone Miner Res*, 16, 782–7.

13   Bauer, D.C. *et al.*, 1992, 'Hyperthyroidism increases the risk of osteoporotic hip fractures. A prospective study', *Journal of Bone and Mineral Research*, 7, S121.

14   Drezner, K., 2004, 'Treatment of anticonvulsant drug-induced bone disease', *Epilepsy Behav*, 5, Suppl 2, S41–7.

15   Pack, A.M. and Morrell, M.J., 2004, 'Epilepsy and bone health in adults', *Epilepsy Behav*, 5, Suppl 2, S24–9.

16   Klotzbuecher, C.M. *et al.*, 2000, 'Patients with prior fractures have an increased risk of future fractures: a summary of the literature and statistical synthesis'. *J Bone Miner Res.*, 15, 721–39.

17   Grainge, M.J. *et al.*, 2001, 'Reproductive, menstrual and menopausal factors: which are associated with bone mineral density in early postmenopausal women?', *Osteoporosis Int.*, 12, 9, 777–87.

Chapter 3

1   Kanis, J.A. and Gluer, C.C., 2000, 'An update on the diagnosis and assessment of osteoporosis with densitometry', Committee of Scientific Advisors, International Osteoporosis Foundation, *Osteoporosis International*, 11, 192–202.

2   Stewart, A. and Reid, 2002, D.M., 'Quantitative ultrasound in osteoporosis', *Semin. Musculoskelet. Radiol*, 6, 229–32.

3   Huopio, J. *et al.*, 2004, 'Calcaneal ultrasound predicts early postmenopausal fractures as well as axial BMD. A prospective study of 422 women', *Osteoporosis International*, 15, 3, 190-5.

4   Gluer, C.C. *et al.*, 2004, 'Association of five quantitative ultrasound devices and bone densitometry with osteoporotic vertebral fractures in a population-based sample: The Opus Study', *J Bone Miner Res*, 19, 5, 782–3.

5   Eastell, R. and Bainbridge, P., 2001, 'Bone turnover markers for monitoring antiresorptive therapy', *Osteoporosis Review*, 9, 1, 1–5.

6   Delmas, P.D. *et al.*, 2000, 'The use of biochemical markers of bone turnover in osteoporosis', Committee of Scientific Advisors, International Osteoporosis Foundation, *Osteoporosis Int.*,(Suppl 6), S2–17.

7   Eastell *et al.*, 'Antifracture efficacy of risedronate: predictions by change in bone resorption markers', Programme and abstracts from Twenty-Third Annual Meeting of the American Society for Bone and Mineral Research, 12–16 October, 2001, Phoenix, Arizona, Abstract 1107. *J Bone Miner Res.* 16 (suppl 1), S163.

8   Xiaoge, D. *et al.*, 2000, 'Bone mineral density differences at the femoral neck and Ward's triangle: a comparison study on the reference data between Chinese and Caucasian women', *Calcif Tissue Int*, 67, 195–8.

9   Wilkins, T.J., 1999, 'Changing perceptions in osteoporosis', *British Medical Journal*, 318, 862–65.

10 Siris, E.S., *et al.*, 2004, 'Bone mineral density thresholds for pharmacological intervention to prevent fractures', *Arch Intern Med*, 164, 10, 1108–12.

11 World Health Organisation,1994, *Assessment of fracture risk and its application to screening for post-menopausal osteoporosis*, WHO, Geneva (Technical report series 843).

12 McClung, M.R. *et al.*, 2001, 'Effect of risedronate treatment on vertebral and non-vertebral fractures with postmenopausal osteoporosis', NEJM, 344-340.

Chapter 4

1   Dawson-Hughes, B. *et al.,* 1997, 'Effect of calcium and vitamin D supplementation on bone density in men and women 65 years of age or older', *New England Journal of Medicine*, 337, 670–6.

2   Mosekilde, L. *et al.,* 2000, 'Hormonal replacement therapy reduces forearm fracture incidence in recent postmenopausal women: results of the Danish Osteoporosis Prevention Study', *Maturitas*, 36, 181–193.

3   Greenspan, S.L. *et al.*, 2002, 'Significant differential effects of alendronate, oestrogen or combination therapy on the rate of bone loss after discontinuation of treatment of postmenopausal osteoporosis: a randomised, double-blind, placebo-controlled trial', *Ann Intern Med*, 137, 875–83.

4   Hoover, R. *et al.,* 1976, 'Menopausal oestrogens and breast cancer', *New England Journal of Medicine*, 295, 401–5.

5   Roussuow, J.E. *et al.*, (Writing Group for the Women's Health Initiative Investigators), 2002, 'Risks and benefits of oestrogen plus progestin in healthy postmenopausal women: principal results from the Women's Health Initiative randomised controlled trial', *Journal of the American Medical Association*, 288, 321–3.

6   Million Women Study Collaborators, 2003, 'Breast cancer and hormone replacement therapy in the Million Women Study', *Lancet*, 362, 419–27.

7   Devogelaer, J.P., 2004, 'A review of the effects of tibolone on the skeleton', *Expert Opin Parmacother*, 5, 4, 941–9.

8   Grady, D. and Cummings, S.R., 2001, 'Postmenopausal hormone therapy for prevention of fractures: how good is the evidence?' *Journal of the American Medical Association*, 285, 22, 2909–10.

9   Willhite, S.L. *et al.*, 1998, 'Raloxifene provides an alternative for osteoporosis prevention', *Ann Pharmacother*, 32, 834–37.

10 Ettinger, B. *et al.*, 1999, 'Reduction of vertebral fracture risk in postmenopausal women with osteoporosis treated with raloxifene: results from a 3 year randomised clinical trial', Multiple Outcomes of Raloxifene Evaluation (MORE) Investigators, *Journal of the American Medical Association*, 282, 637–45.

11 Kanis J.A. *et al.*, 2003, 'Effect of raloxifene on the risk of new vertebral fracture in postmenopausal women with osteopenia or osteoporosis: a reanalysis of the Multiple Outcomes of Raloxifene Evaluation trial', *Bone*, 33, 3, 293–300.

12   Layton, D. *et al.*, 2004, 'Safety profile of raloxifene as used in general practice in England: results of a prescription-event monitoring study, *Osteoporosis Int*, 7 August.

13 Storm, T. *et al.*, 1990, 'Effect of intermittent cyclical etidronate therapy on bone mass, fracture rate in women with postmenopausal osteoporosis', *New England Journal of Medicine*, 322, 1265–71.

14 Lin, J.H., 1996, 'Bisphosphonates: a review of their pharmacokinetic properties', *Bone*, 18, 75–85.

15 Hosking, D. *et al.*, 1998, 'Prevention of bone loss with alendronate in postmenopausal women under 60 years of age', *New England Journal of Medicine*, 338, 485–92.

16 Black, D.M. *et al.*, 1996, 'Randomised trial of effect of alendronate on risk of fracture in women with existing vertebral fractures', Fracture Intervention Trial Research Group, *Lancet*, 348, 1535–41 and Cummings, S.R. *et al.*, 1998, 'Effect of alendronate on risk of fracture in women with low bone density but without vertebral fractures: results from the Fracture Intervention Trial', *JAMA*, 280, 2077–82.

17   Harris, S.T. *et al.*, 1999, 'Effects of risedronate treatment on vertebral and nonvertebral fractures in women with postmenopausal osteoporosis: a randomised controlled trial', Vertebral Efficacy with Risedronate Therapy (VERT) Study Group, *Journal of the American Medical Association*, 282, 1344–52.

18 Strewler, G.J., 2004, 'Decimal point – osteoporosis therapy at the ten year mark', *NEJM*, 350, 12, 1172–4.

19 Ott, S.M., 2001, 'Fractures after long-term alendronate therapy', *J Clin Endocrinol Metabol*, 86, 4, 1835.

20 Tonino, R.P. *et al.*, 2000, 'Skeletal benefits of alendronate seven year treatment of postmenopausal osteoporotic women', *J Clin Endocrinol Metabol*, 85, 3109–15.

21 Bone, H.G. *et al.*, 2004, 'Ten years' experience with alendronate for osteoporosis in postmenopausal women', *NEJM*, 350, 12, 1189–99.

22 Reginster, J.Y. *et al.*, 2000, 'Randomised trial of the effects of risedronate on vertebral fractures in women with established postmenopausal osteoporosis', *Osteoporosis Int*, 11, 83–91.

23 Kanis, J.A. and McCloskey, E.V., 1999, 'Effect of calcitonin on vertebral and other fractures', *Q J Med*, 92, 143–9.

24 Neer, R.M., 2001, 'Effect of parathyroid hormone (1-34) on fractures and bone mineral density in postmenopausal women with osteoporosis', *NEJM*, 344, 1434–41.

25 FDA Talk Paper, 26 November, 2002.

26 Meunier, P.J., 2004, 'The effects of strontium ranelate on the risk of vertebral fracture in women with postmenopausal osteoporosis', *NEJM*, 350, 459–68.

27 Reginster, J.Y. *et al.*, 2002, 'Strontium ranelate reduces the risk of hip fracture in women with postmenopausal osteoporosis', *Osteo Int*, 13, S14.

28 Lee, J.R., 1990, 'Osteoporosis reversal, the role of progesterone', *Int Clin Nutr Rev*, 10, 3.

29 Leonetti, H.B. *et al*, 1999, ;Transdermal progesterone cream for vasomotor symptoms and postmenopausal bone loss', *Obstet Gynaecol*, 94, 2, 225–8.

30 Solomon, D.H. *et al.*, 2004, 'Statin lipid-lowering drugs and bone mineral density', *Pharmacoepidemiol Drug Saf*, 20 July.

31 Rejnmark, L. *et al.*, 2004, 'Effects of simvastatin on bone turnover and BMD: A 1-year randomised controlled trial in postmenopausal osteopenic women', *J Bone Miner Res*, 19, 5, 737–44.

32 Bauer, D.C. *et al.*, 2004, 'Use of statins and fracture: results of 4 prospective studies and cumulative meta-analysis of observational studies and controlled trials', *Arch Intern Med*, 164, 2, 146–52.

33 Ascer, E. *et al.*, 2004, 'Atorvastatin reduces proinflammatory markers in hypercholesterolemic patients', *Atherosclerosis*, 177, 1, 161–6.

34 Goodman G.D., 1992, 'Interleukin-6: An osteotropic factor?', *J Bone Miner Res*, 7, 475–6.

35 Rundek, T. *et al.*, 2004, 'Atorvastin decreases the coenzyme Q10 level in the blood of patients at risk of cardiovascular disease and stroke', *Arch Neurol*, 61, 6, 889–92.

36 Langsjoen, P.H. *et al.*, 1990, 'A six year clinical study of therapy of cardiomyopathy with coenzyme Q10', *Int J Tissue React*, 12, 3, 169–71.

37 Berman, M. *et al.*, 2004, 'Coenzyme Q10 in patients with end-stage heart failure awaiting cardiac transplantation: a randomised, placebo-controlled study', *Clin Cardiol*, 27, 5, 295–9.

38 Sacks, F.M., 1996, 'The effects of pravastatin on coronary events after myocardial infarction in patients with average cholesterol levels', Cholesterol and Recurrent Events (CARE) Trial Investigators, *NEJM*, 335, 1001–9.

39 Friis, S. *et al.*, 2004, 'Cancer risk among statin users: A population-based cohort study', *Int J Cancer*, December.

40 Rundek, T. *et al*, 2004, 'Atorvastin decreases the coenzyme Q10 level in the blood of patients at risk of cardiovascular disease and stroke', Arch Neurol, 61, 6, 889–92.

41 Kurttio, P. *et al.*, 1999, 'Exposure to natural fluoride in well water and hip fracture: a cohort analysis in Finland', *American Journal of Epidemiology*, 150, 817–24.

42 Kaunitz, A.M., 2003, 'Osteopenia in a premenopausal woman', *Ob Gyn and Women's Health*, 8, 1.

43 Gourlay, M.L. and Brown, S.A., 2004, 'Clinical considerations in premenopausal osteoporosis', *Arch Intern Med*, 164, 603–14.

Chapter 5

1   Frassetto, L.A. *et al.*, 1996, 'Effect of age on blood acid-base composition in adult humans: role of age-related renal functional decline', *Am J Physiol*, (Renal Fluid Electrolyte Physiol, 40), 271, F1114–22.

2   Kerstetter, J.E. *et al.*, 1999, 'Changes in bone turnover in young women consuming different levels of dietary protein', *Journal of Clinical Endocrinology and Metabolism*, 84, 1052–5.

3   Kersetteer, J.E. and Allen, L.H., 1989, 'Dietary protein increases urine calcium', *American Institute of Nutrition*, 120, 134–6.

4   Clifton, P.M. *et al.*, 2003, 'Effect of an energy reduced high protein red meat diet on weight loss and metabolic parameters in obese women', *Asia Pac J Clin Nutr*, 12, S10 and Farnsworth, E. *et al.*, 2003, 'Effect of a high protein, energy restricted diet on body composition, glycemic control and lipid concentrations in overweight and obese hyperinsulinemic men and women', *Am J Clin Nutr*, 78, 1, 31–9.

5   Sellmeyer, D.E. *et al.*, 2001, 'A high ratio of dietary animal to vegetable protein increases the rate of bone loss and the risk of fracture in postmenopausal women', Study of Osteoporotic Fractures Research Group, *Am J Clin Nutr*, 73, 1, 118–22.

6   Feskanich, *et al.*, 1996, 'Protein Consumption and Bone Fractures in Women', *American Journal of Epidemiology*, 143, 5, 472–9.

7   Frassetto, L.A. *et al.*, 2000, 'Worldwide incidence of hip fractures in elderly women: relation to consumption of animal and vegetable foods', *J Gerontol A Biol Sci Med Sci*, 55, 10, M585–92.

8   From Frassetto. L.A. *et al.*, 2000, 'Worldwide incidence of hip fractures in elderly women: relation to consumption of animal and vegetable foods', *J Gerontol A Biol Sci Med Sci*, 55, 10, M585–92.

9   Sanchez, V. *et al.*, 1978, 'Bone mineral mass in elderly vegetarian females', *American Journal of Roentgenol*, 131, 542.

10 Ellis, F *et al.*, 1972, 'Incidence of osteoporosis in vegetarians and omnivores', *American Journal of Clinical Nutrition*, 25, 55–8.

11 Reed, J.A. *et al.*, 1994, 'Comparative changes in radial bone density of elderly female lactoovovegetarians and omnivores', *American Journal of Clinical Nutrition*, 59, 1197S–202S.

12 Marsh, A.G. *et al.*, 1988, 'Vegetarian lifestyle and bone mineral density', *American Journal of Clinical Nutrition*, 48, 837–41.

13 Harvard School of Public Health, 2004.

14 Larsson, S.C., 2004, 'Milk and lactose intakes and ovarian cancer risk in the Swedish Mammography Cohort', *American Journal of Clinical Nutrition*, 80, 5, 1353–7.

15 Du, XQ *et al.*, 2002, 'Milk consumption and bone mineral content in Chinese adolescent girls', *Bone*, 30, 521–8.

16 Fleming, K.H. *et al.*, 1994, 'Consumption of calcium in the US: food sources and intake levels', *J Nutr*, 124, 1426S–30S.

17 Ho, S.C. *et al.*, 1994, 'Determinants of bone mass in Chinese women aged 21-40 years. II. Pattern of dietary calcium intake and association with bone mineral density', *Osteo Int*, 4, 167–75.

18 Xiaoge, D. *et al.*, 2000, 'Bone mineral density differences at the femoral neck and Ward's triangle: a comparison study on the reference data between Chinese and Caucasian women', *Calcif Tissue Int*, 67, 195–8.

19 Fujita, T. and Fukase, M., 1992, 'Comparison of osteoporosis and calcium intake between Japan and the United States', *Proc Soc Exp Biol Med*, 200, 2, 149–52.

20 Ho, S.C. *et al.*, 1993, 'Hip fracture rates in Hong Kong and the United States', 1988 through 1989, *Am J Public Health*, 83, 694–7.

21 Remer, T. and Manz, F., 1995, 'Potential renal acid load of foods and its influence on urine pH', *J Am Diet Assoc*, 95, 791–7.

22 Remer, T. and Manz, F., 1995, 'Potential renal acid load of foods and its influence on urine pH', *J Am Diet Assoc*, 95, 791–7.

23 Information taken from Remer, T. and Manz, F., 1995, 'Potential renal acid load of foods and its influence on urine pH', *J Am Diet Assoc*, 95, 791–7.

24 Remer, T. and Manz, F., 1995, 'Potential renal acid load of foods and its influence on urine pH', *J Am Diet Assoc*, 95, 791–7.

25 Frassetto, L. *et al.*, 2001, 'Diet evolution and ageing – the pathophysiologic effects of the postagricultural inversion of the potassium-to-sodium and base-chloride ratios in the human diet', *Eur J Nutr*, 40, 200–13.

26 Muhlabauer, R.C. *et al.*, 2002, 'Onion and a mixture of vegetables, salads and herbs affect bone resorption in the rat by a mechanism independent of their base excess', *J Bone Miner Res*.

27 Massey, L.K. and Whiting, S.J., 1996, 'Dietary salt, urinary calcium and bone loss', *J Bone Miner Res*, 11, 731–6.

28 Sellmeyer, D.E. *et al.*, 2001, 'A high ratio of dietary animal to vegetable protein increases the rate of bone loss and the risk of fracture in postmenopausal women', Study of Osteoporotic Fractures Research Group, *American Journal of Clinical Nutrition*, 73, 1, 118–22.

29 Sebastian, A. *et al.*, 1994, 'Improved mineral balance and skeletal metabolism in postmenopausal women treated with potassium bicarbonate', *NEJM*, 330, 25, 1776-81.

30 Ronco, *et al.*, 1999, 'Vegetables, fruits and related nutrients and risk of breast cancer: a case-control study in Uruguay', *Nutr Cancer*, 35, 111–19.

31 Law and Morris, 1998, 'By how much does fruit and vegetable consumption reduce the risk of ischaemic heart disease', *Eur J Clin Nutr*, 52, 549–56.

32 Remer, T. and Manz, F., 1995, 'Potential renal acid load of foods and its influence on urine pH', *J Am Diet Assoc*, 95, 791–7.

33 US Department of Agriculture, 2004.

34 Hansen, S.A. *et al.*, 2000, 'Association of fractures with caffeine and alcohol in postmenopausal women, the Iowa Women's Health Study', *Public Health Nutr*, 3, 253–61.

35 Holbrook, T.L. and Barrett-Conner, E., 1993, 'A prospective study of alcohol consumption and bone mineral density', *British Medical Journal*, 1056–8.

36 Al-Masri, B.K. *et al.*, 2002, Second Pan-Arab Osteoporosis Congress, Third International Congress of the Egyptian Osteoporosis Prevention Society, Sharm El Sheikh, Egypt, 22–25 October.

37 Rapuri, P.B. *et al.*, 2001, 'Caffeine intake increases the rate of bone loss in elderly women and interacts with vitamin D receptor genotypes', *American Journal of Clinical Nutrition*, 74, 5, 694–700.

38 Hegarty, V. *et al.*, 2000, 'Tea drinking and bone mineral density in older women'. *American Journal of Clinical Nutrition*, 71, 1003–7.

39 Basu, S. *et al.*, 2001, 'Association between oxidative stress and bone mineral density', *Biochem Biophys Res Commun*, 288, 1, 275–9.

40 Massey, L.K. and Hollingbery, P.W., 1988, 'Acute effects of dietary caffeine and sucrose on urinary mineral excretion of healthy adolescent', *Nutr Res*, 8, 1005–12.

41 Hannan, M.T. *et al.*, 2000, 'Risk factors for longitudinal bone loss in elderly men and women: the Framingham Osteoporosis Study', *J Bone Miner Res*, 15, 710–20.

42 Saffar, J.L. *et al.*, 1981, 'Osteoporotic effect of a high carbohydrate diet in golden hamsters', *Arch Oral Biol*, 26, 393–7.

43 Ringsdorf, W. *et al.*, 1976, 'Sucrose, neutrophil phagocytosis and resistance to disease', *Dent Surv*, 52, 46–8.

44 Budd, M., 1995, *Low Blood Sugar*, Thorsons.

45 Blundell, J.E. and Hill, A.J. 1986, 'Paradoxical effects of an intense sweetener (aspartame) on appetite', *Lancet*, 1, 1092–3.

46 Wurtman, R.J. 1983, 'Neurochemical changes following high dose aspartame with dietary carbohydrates', *New England Journal of Medicine*, 429–30.

47 Stegink, L.D. *et al.*, 1989, 'Effect of repeated ingestion of aspartame-sweetened beverage on plasma amino acid, blood methanol and blood formate concentrations', *Metabolism*, 38, 4, 357–63.

48 Lipton, S.A. and Rosenberg. P.A., 1994, 'Excitatory amino acids as a final common pathway for neurologic disorders', *New England Journal of Medicine*, 300, 9, 613–22.

49 Barzel, U.S. and Massey, L.K., 1998, 'Excess dietary protein can adversely affect bone', *J Nutr*, 128, 1051–3.

50 Brown, S., 2000, 'Acid-alkaline balance and its effect on bone health', *International Journal of Integrative Medicine*, 2, 6.

51 Wyshak, G., 2000, 'Teenage girls, carbonated beverages and bone fractures', *Arch Pediatr Adolesc Med*, 154, 610–13.

52 Goldsmith, *et al.*, 1976, 'Effects of phosphorus supplementation on serum parathyroid hormone and bone morphology in osteoporosis', *Journal of Clinical Endocrin Metab*, 523–32).

53 American Academy of Pediatrics, Policy Statement, 2004, 'Soft drinks in school', *Pediatrics*, 113, 1, 152–4.

54 Rico, H., 1990, 'Alcohol and bone disease', *Alcohol Alcohol*, 25, 345–52.

55 Felson, D. *et al.*, 1988, 'Alcohol consumption and hip fractures: the Framingham study', *American Journal of Epidemiology*, 128, 1102–10.

56 Rapuri, P.B. *et al.*, 2000, 'Alcohol intake and bone metabolism in elderly women', *American Journal of Clinical Nutrition*, 72, 1206–13.

57 Goulding, A., 1990, 'Osteoporosis: why consuming less sodium chloride helps to conserve bone', *New Zealand Medical Journal*, 102, 12–122.

58 Nordin, B.E.C. *et al.*, 1993, 'The nature and significance of the relationship between urinary sodium and urinary calcium in women', *J Nutr*, 123, 1615–22.

59 Cappuccio, F.P. *et al.*, 1999, 'High blood pressure and bone mineral density in elderly white women: a prospective study', Study of Osteoporotic Fractures Research Group, *Lancet*, 354, 9183, 971–5.

60 Lemann, L. *et al.*, 1989, 'Potassium bicarbonate, but not sodium bicarbonate, reduces urinary calcium excretion and improves calcium balance in healthy men', *Kidney Int*, 35, 688–95.

61 Greendale, G.A. *et al.*, 1999, 'The relation between cortisol excretion and fractures in healthy older people: results from the MacArthur Studies', *J Am Geriatr Soc*, 47, 799–803.

62 Tylvasky, F.A., 2002, 'Fruit and vegetable intake is an independent predictor of bone mass in early-pubertal children', *J Bone Miner Res*, 17, S459.

63 New, S.A. *et al.*, 2000, 'Dietary influences on bone mass and bone metabolism: further evidence of a positive link between fruit and vegetable consumption and bone health?', *American Journal of Clinical Nutrition*, 71, 142–51.

64 New, S.A. *et al.*, 2000, 'Dietary influences on bone mass and bone metabolism: further evidence of a positive link between fruit and vegetable consumption and bone health?', *American Journal of Clinical Nutrition*, 71, 142–51.

65 Tucker, K.L. *et al.*, 1999, 'Potassium and fruit and vegetables are associated with greater bone mineral density in elderly men and women', *American Journal of Clinical Nutrition*, 69, 727–36.

66 Arnett, T.R. and Spowage, M., 1996, 'Modulation of the resorptive activity of rat osteoclasts by small changes in extracellular pH near the physiological range', *Bone*, 18, 277–9.

67 Kerstetter, J.E. *et al.*, 2003, 'Dietary protein, calcium metabolism and skeletal homeostasis revisited', *American Journal of Clinical Nutrition*, 78, 3 Suppl, 584S–592S.

68 Kishi M. *et al.*, 1999, 'Enhancing effect of dietary vinegar on the intestinal absorption of calcium in ovariectomised rats', *Bioscience, Biotechnology and Biochemistry*, 63, 5, 905–10.

69 Kessel, B., 1996, 'Alternatives to oestrogen for menopausal women', *Proc Soc Exp Biol Med*, 217, 38–44.

70 Boulet, M., 1994, 'Climacteric and menopause in seven south-east Asian countries', *Maturitas*, 19, 157–76.

71 Brezinski, 1999, 'Phytoestrogens, the "natural" SERMS?', *Eur J Obs Gynae*, 85, 47–51.
72 Hall, J.M. and McDoriesnnell, D.P., 1999, 'The oestrogen receptor beta-isoform (ERbeta) of the human oestrogen receptor modulates ERalpha transcriptional activity and is a key regulator of the cellular response to oestrogens and antioestrogens', *Endocrinology*, 140, 12, 5566–78.
73 Coleman, M.P. *et al.*, 1993, *Trends in Cancer Incidence and Mortality*, Lyon, France, IARC Publication, 1213, presented at the European Society for Therapeutic Radiology and Oncology, 1996.
74 Cumming, R.S. and Menton, III, L.J., 2002, 'Epidemiology and outcome of osteoporosis fractures', *Lancet*, 1761–7.
75 Somekawa, Y. *et al.*, 2001, 'Soy intake related to menopausal symptoms, serum lipids and bone mineral density in postmenopausal Japanese women', *Obstetrics and Gynaecology*, 97, 1, 109–15.
76 Phillimore, Jane, 2000, 'Soya Bean Crisis', *Observer* magazine, 27 August.
77 Lappe, M.A. *et al.*, 1999, 'Alterations in clinically important phytoestrogens in genetically modified, herbicide-tolerant soybeans', *Journal of Medicinal Food*, 1, 4.
78 Kessler, T. and Hesse, A., 2000, 'Cross-over study of the influence of bicarbonate-rich mineral water on urinary composition in comparison with sodium potassium citrate in healthy male subjects', *Br J Nutr*, 84, 865–71.
79 Bohmer, H. *et al.*, 2000, 'Calcium supplementation with calcium-rich mineral waters: a systematic review and meta-analysis of its bioavailability', *Osteoporosis Int*, 11, 938–43.
80 Halpern, G.M. *et al.*, 1991, 'Comparative uptake of calcium from milk and a calcium-rich mineral water in lactose intolerant adults: implications for treatment of osteoporosis', *Am J Prev Med*, 7, 6, 379–83.

Chapter 6

1 Markovic, V. *et al.*, 1995, 'Calcium intake and skeletal formation', *Challenges Mod Med*, 7, 129–45.
2 Shea, B. *et al.*, 2002, 'Meta-analysis of calcium supplementation for the prevention of postmenopausal osteoporosis', *Endocrine Rev*, 23, 4, 552–529.
3 Shea B. *et al.*, 2004, 'Calcium supplementation on bone loss in postmenopausal women', *Cochrane Database Syst Rev*, 1, CD004526.
4 Shea, B. *et al.*, 2000, 'A meta-analysis of calcium supplementation for the prevention of postmenopausal osteoporosis', *Osteoporosis International*, 11, S114.
5 Dawson-Hughes, B. *et al.*, 2000, 'Effect of withdrawal of calcium and vitamin D supplements on bone mass in elderly men and women', *American Journal of Clinical Nutrition*, 72, 3, 745–50.
6 Calvo, M.S. *et al.*, 1991, 'Circadian variation in ionised calcium and intact parathyroid hormone: evidence for sex differences in calcium homeostasis', *J Clin Endocrinol Metabol*, 72, 1, 69–76.

7   Sakhaee, K. *et al.*, 1999, 'Meta-analysis of calcium bioavailability: a comparison of calcium citrate and calcium carbonate', *American Journal of Therapeutics*, 5, 313–21.

8   Carr, C.J. and Shangraw, R.F., 1987, 'Nutritional and pharmaceutical aspects of calcium supplementation', *Am Pharm*, 27, 49–57.

9   Hegsted, D.M., 2001, 'Fractures, calcium and the modern diet', *American Journal of Clinical Nutrition*, 74, 5, 571–3.

10 Prentice, A. *et al.*, 1991, 'Bone mineral content of British and rural Gambian women aged 18–80+ years', *Bone Mineral*, 12, 3, 201–14.

11 Damien, D., 2001, 'Vitamin D - Time for Reassessment', *Journal of Nutritional and Environmental Medicine*, 11, 237–9.

12 Nowson, C.A. and Magerison, C., 2002, 'Vitamin D intake and vitamin D status of Australians', *Med J Aust*, 177, 3, 149–52.

13 Heikinheimo, R.J. *et al.*, 1992, 'Annual injection of vitamin D and fractures of aged bones', *Calcif Tissue Int*, 51, 105–10.

14 Plotnikoff, G.A. and Quigley, J.M., 2003, 'Prevalence of severe hypovitaminosis D in patients with persistent, non-specific musculoskeletal pain', *Mayo Clin Proc*, 78, 12, 1463–70.

15 Al Faraj, S. *et al.*, 2003, 'Vitamin D deficiency and chronic low back pain in Saudi Arabia', *Spine*, 28, 2, 177–9.

16 Chapuy, M.C. *et al.*, 1994, 'Effect of calcium and cholecalciferol treatment for three years on hip fracture in elderly women', *British Medical Journal*, 308, 1081–2.

17 Dawson-Hughes, B. *et al.*, 2000, 'Effect of withdrawal of calcium and vitamin D supplements on bone mass in elderly men and women', *American Journal of Clinical Nutrition*, 72, 745–50.

18 Trang, H.M. *et al.*, 1998, 'Evidence that vitamin D3 increases serum 25-hydroxyvitamin D more efficiently than does vitamin D', *American Journal of Clinical Nutrition*, 68, 854–858.

19 Humphries *et al.*, 1999, 'Low dietary magnesium is associated with insulin resistance in a sample of young non-diabetic Black Americans', *Am J Hypertension*, 12, 747–56.

20 Rude, R.K., 1998, 'Magnesium Deficiency: a heterogeneous cause of disease in humans', *J Bone Miner Res*, 13, 749–58.

21 New, S.A. *et al.*, 1997, 'Nutritional influences on bone mineral density: a cross-sectional study in premenopausal women', *American Journal of Clinical Nutrition*, 65, 1831–9.

22 Wang, M.C. *et al.*, 1999, 'Influence of pre-adolescent diet on quantitative ultrasound measurements of the calcaneus in young adult women', *Osteoporosis Int*, 9, 532–5.

23 Current Research in Osteoporosis and Bone Mineral Measurement II, British Institute of Radiology, 1992.

24 Sojka, J.E., 1995, 'Magnesium supplementation and osteoporosis', *Nutrition Reviews*, 53, 71–80.

25 Creedon, A. *et al.*, 1999, 'The effect of moderately and severely restricted dietary magnesium intakes on bone composition and bone metabolism in the rate', *British Journal of Nutrition*, 82, 63–71.

26 Stending-Lindberg, G. *et al.*, 1993, 'Trabecular bone density in a two year controlled trial of personal magnesium in osteoporosis', *Magnesium Research*, 6, 155–63.

27 Faccinetti, F. *et al.*, 1991, 'Magnesium prophylaxis of menstrual migraine: effects on intracellular magnesium', *Headache*, 31, 298–304.

28 Blackburn, G.L., 2004,' A new risk factor for fractures? Diets low in B vitamins may leave people more prone to broken bones', *Health News*, 10, 7, 12.

29 Stone, K.L. *et al.*, 2004, 'Low serum vitamin B12 levels are associated with increased hip bone loss in older women: a prospective study', *J Clin Endocrinol Metab*, 89, 3, 1217–21.

30 van Meurs, J.B.J. *et al.*, 2004, 'Homocysteine levels and risk of osteoporotic fracture', *NEJM*, 350, 2033–41 and McLean, R.R. *et al.*, 2004, 'Homocysteine as a predictive factor for hip fracture in older persons', *NEJM*, 350, 2042–9.

31 Feskanich, D. *et al.*, 1999, 'Dietary vitamin K and hip fractures in women: a prospective study', *American Journal of Clinical Nutrition*, 69, 1, 74–9.

32 Booth, S.L. and Suttie, J.W., 1999, 'Dietary intake and adequacy of vitamin K', *J Nutr*, 128, 5, 785–88.

33 Braam, L.A. *et al.*, 2003, 'Vitamin K supplementation retards bone loss in postmenopausal women between 50 and 60 years of age', *Calcif Tissue Int*, 73, 21–6.

34 Shearer, M.J. *et al.*, 1996, 'Chemistry, nutritional sources, tissue distribution and metabolism of vitamin K with special reference to bone health', *Journal of Nutrition*, 126, 1181S–6S.

35 Neilsen, F.H. *et al.*, 1987, 'Effect of dietary boron on mineral, oestrogen and testosterone metabolism in postmenopausal women', *FASEB J*, 1, 394–7.

36 Calhoun, N.R. *et al.*, 1975, 'The effects of zinc on ectopic bone formation', *Oral Surg* 39, 698–706.

37 Herzberg, M. *et al.*, 1996, 'The effect of oestrogen replacement therapy on zinc in serum and urine', *Obstet Gynaecol*, 87, 145–54.

38 Angus, R.M. *et al.*, 1988, 'Dietary intake and bone mineral density', *Clin Nutr*, 46, 2, 265–77.

39 Freudenheim, J.L., 1986, 'Relationship between usual nutrient intake and bone mineral content of women 35-65 years of age: longitudinal and cross sectional analysis', *American Journal of Clinical Nutrition*, 44, 863–76.

40 Kruger, M.C. 1998, 'Calcium, gamma-linolenic acid and eicosapentaenoic acid supplementation in senile osteoporosis', *Ageing* (Milano), 10, 385–94.

41 Sakaguchi, K. *et al.*, 1994, 'Prostaglandins Leukotrienes EFAs', 50, 81–4.

42 Lippiello, L. and Feinhold, M., 1993, *Arthritis Rheum*, 36, 5165.

43 Lim, L.S. *et al.*, 2004, 'Vitamin A intake and the risk of hip fracture in postmenopausal women: the Iowa women's health study', *Osteoporosis Int*, 3 February.

44 Feskanich, D. *et al.*, 2002, 'Vitamin A intake and hip fractures among postmenopausal women', *Journal of the American Medical Association*, 287, 1, 47–54.

45 Setchell, K.D. and Lydeking-Olsen, E., 2003, 'Dietary phytoestrogens and their effect on bone: evidence from in vitro and in vivo, human observational and dietary intervention studies', *American Journal of Clinical Nutrition*, 78 (3 Suppl), 593S–609S.

46 Ishida, H. *et al.*, 1998, 'Preventative effects of the plant isoflavones, daidzein and genistein, on bone loss in ovariectomised rats fed a calcium-deficient diet', *Biol, Pharm. Bull*, 21, 62–6.

47 Picherit, C. *et al.*, 2001, 'Soybean isoflavones dose-dependently reduce bone turnover but do not reverse established osteopenia in adult ovariectomised rats', *J Nutr*, 131, 723-281.

48 Gallagher, J.C. *et al.*, 2004, 'The effect of soya protein isolate on bone metabolism', *Menopause*, 11, 3, 290–8.

49 Schreiber, M.D. and Rebar, R.W.F., 1999, 'Isoflavones and postmenopausal bone health: a viable alternative to oestrogen therapy', *Menopause*, 6, 3, 233–41.

50 Halpner, A.D. *et al.*, 2000, 'The effect of an ipriflavone-containing supplement on urinary N-linked telopeptide levels in postmenopausal women', *Women's Health Gend Based Med*, 9, 995–8.

51 Atkinson, C. *et al.*, 2004, 'The effects of phytoestrogen isoflavones on bone density in women: a double-blind, randomised, placebo-controlled trial', *American Journal of Clinical Nutrition*, 79, 2, 326–33.

52 Lydeking-Olsen, E. *et al.*, 2004, 'Soymilk or progesterone for prevention of bone loss: A two year randomised, placebo-controlled trial', *Eur J Nutr*, 1–12.

53 Alexandersen, P., 2001, 'Ipriflavone in the treatment of postmenopausal osteoporosis: a randomised controlled trial', Ipriflavone Multicentre European Fracture Study, *Journal of the American Medical Association*, 285, 1482–8.

54 Nisslein, T. and Freudenstein, J., 2003, 'Effects of an isopropanolic extract of Cimicifuga racemosa on urinary crosslinks and other parameters of bone quality in an ovariectomised rat model of osteoporosis', *J Bone Miner Metab*, 21, 6, 370–6.

55 Seidlova-Wuttke, D. *et al.*, 2003, 'Evidence for selective estrogen receptor modulator activity in a black cohosh (Cimicifuga racemosa) extract: comparison with oestradiol-17beta', *Eur J Endocrinol*, 149, 4, 351–62.

Chapter 7

1 Kai, M.C. *et al.*, 2003, 'Exercise interventions: defusing the world's osteoporosis time bomb', *Bulletin of World Health Organisation*, 81, 11, 827–30.

2 Vico, L. *et al.*, 2000, 'Effects of long term microgravity exposure on cancellous and cortical weight-bearing bones of cosmonauts', *The Lancet*, 355, 1607–11.

3 Holick, M.F., 2000, 'Microgravity-induced bone loss – will it limit human space exploration?', *Lancet*, 355, 1569–70.

4 Lee, I.M. *et al.*, 1997, 'Physical activity, physical fitness and longevity', *Ageing* (Milano), 9, 2-11.

5   Bernstein, L., 1994, *Journal of the National Cancer Institute*, 86, 18.

6   Friedenreich, C.M. *et al.*, 2001, 'Influence of physical activity in different age and life periods on the risk of breast cancer', *Epidemiology*, 12, 6, 604–12.

7   Feskanich, D. *et al.*, 2002, 'Walking and leisure-time activity and risk of hip fracture in postmenopausal women', *Journal of the American Medical Association*, 288, 2300–6.

8   Wolfgang, K. *et al.*, 2004, 'Benefits of 2 years of intense exercise on bone density, physical fitness and blood lipids in early postmenopausal osteopenic women', *Arch Intern Med*, 164, 10, 1084–91.

9   Taaffe, D.R. *et al.*, 1995, 'Differential effects of swimming versus weight-bearing activity on bone mineral status of eumenorrheic athletes', *J Bone Min Res*, 586–93.

10   Kohort, W.M. *et al.*, 1997, 'Effects of exercise involving predominantly either joint-reaction or ground-reaction forces on bone mineral density in older women', *J Bone Miner Res*, 12, 1253–61.

11   Bassey, E.J., 2001, 'Exercise for improving bone mineral density: the benefits of weight training', *Osteoporosis Review*, 9, 4, 11–13.

12   Wolf, S.L. *et al.*, 1996, 'Reducing frailty and falls in older persons: an investigation of T'ai Chi and computerised balance training', *J Am Geriatric Soc*, 44, 599–600.

13   Flieger, J. *et al.*, 1998, 'Mechanical stimulation in the form of vibration prevents postmenopausal bone loss in ovariectomised rats', *Calcif Tissue Int*, 63, 510–14).

14   Salamone, L.M. *et al.*, 1999, 'Effect of a lifestyle intervention on bone mineral density in premenopausal women: a randomised trial', *American Journal of Clinical Nutrition*, 70, 1, 97–103.

Chapter 8

1   Pocock, N.A. *et al.*, 1987, 'Genetic determinants of bone mass in adults: a twin study', *J Clin Invest*, 80, 706–10.

2   Zeigler, R.G. *et al.*, 1993, 'Migration patterns and breast cancer risk in Asian-American women', *J Natl Cancer Inst*, 85, 22, 1819–27.

3   Burghes, A.H. *et al.*, 2001, 'The land between Mendelian and multifactorial inheritance', *Science*, 293, 2213–14.

4   Qureshi, A.M. *et al.*, 2002, 'COLIA1 Sp1 polymorphism predicts response of femoral neck bone density to cyclical etidronate therapy', *Calcif Tissue Int*, 70, 158–63.

5   Roses, A.D., 2000, 'Pharmacogenetics and the practice of medicine', *Nature*, 405, 857–86.

6   McGuigan, F.E.A. *et al.*, 2001, 'Prediction of osteoporotic fractures by bone densitometry and COL1A1 genotyping: a prospective, population-based study in men and women', *Osteoporosis Int*, 12, 91–6.

7   Brown, M.A. *et al.*, 2001, 'Genetic control of bone density and turnover: role of the collagen 1alpha1, oestrogen receptor and vitamin D receptor genes', *J Bone Miner Res*, 16, 4, 758–64.

8   Beavan, S. *et al.*, 1998, 'Polymorphism of the collagen type 1 alpha 1 gene and ethnic differences in hip fracture rates', *NEJM*, 339, 351–2.

9   Taboulet, J. *et al.*, 1998, 'Calcitonin receptor polymorphism is associated with a decreased fracture risk in postmenopausal women', *Hum Mol Genet*, 7, 13, 2129–33.

10 Cooper, G.S. *et al.*, 1996, 'Are vitamin D receptor polymorphisms associated with bone mineral density? A meta-analysis', *J Bone Miner Res*, 11, 12, 1841–9.

11 Morrison, N.A. *et al.*, 1992, 'Contribution of trans-acting factor alleles to normal physiological variability: vitamin D receptor gene polymorphism and circulating osteocalcin', *Proc Natl Acad Sci*, 89, 15, 6665–9.

12 Feskanich, D. *et al.*, 1998, 'Vitamin D receptor site genotype and the risk of bone fractures in women', *Epidemiology*, 9, 535–9.

13 Peacock, M., 1995, 'Vitamin D receptor gene alleles and osteoporosis: a contrasting view', *J Bone Miner Res*, 10, 1294–7.

14 Krall, E.A. *et al.*, 1995, 'Vitamin D receptor alleles and rates of bone loss: incidence of years since menopause and calcium intake', *J Bone Miner Res*, 10, 978–84.

15 Rapuri, P.B. *et al.*, 2001, 'Caffeine intake increases the rate of bone loss in elderly women and interacts with vitamin D receptor genotypes', *American Journal of Clinical Nutrition*, 74, 5, 694–700.

16 Robsahm, T.E. *et al.*, 2004, 'Vitamin D3 from sunlight may improve the prognosis of breast, colon and prostate cancer', *Cancer Causes Control*, 15, 2, 149–58.

17 Guy, M. *et al.*, 2004, 'Vitamin D receptor gene polymorphisms and breast cancer risk', *Clin Cancer Res*, 10, 16, 5472–81.

18 Silanpaa, P. *et al.*, 2004, 'Vitamin D receptor gene polymorphism as an important modifier of positive family history related breast cancer risk', *Pharmacogenetics*, 14, 4, 239–45.

19 Goodman, G.D., 1992, 'Interleukin-6: An osteotropic factor?', *J Bone Miner Res*, 7, 475–6.

20 Jilka, R.L., 1998, 'Cytokines, bone remodelling and oestrogen deficiency', *Bone*, 23, 75–81.

21 Murray, R.E. *et al.*, 1997, 'Polymorphisms of the interleukin-6 gene are associated with bone mineral density', *Bone*, 21, 89–92.

22 Spotila, L.D. *et al.*, 2000, 'Association of a polymorphism in the TNFR2 gene with low bone mineral density', *J Bone Miner Res*, 15, 1376–83.

23 Pfleilschifler, J. *et al.*, 2002, 'Changes in pro-inflammatory cytokine activity after menopause', *Endocrine Reviews*, 23, 90.

24 Weel, A.E. *et al.*, 1999, 'Oestrogen receptor polymorphism predicts the onset of natural and surgical menopause', *J Clin Endocrinol Metab*, 84, 3146–50.

25 Becherini, L. *et al.*, 2000, 'Evidence of a linkage disequilibrium between polymorphisms in the human oestrogen receptor alpha gene and their

relationship to bone mass variation in postmenopausal Italian Women', *Human Mol Genet*, 9, 2043–50.

27 Ioannidis, J.P. *et al.*, 2004, 'Differential genetic effects of ESR1 gene polymorphisms on osteoporosis outcomes', *Journal of the American Medical Association*, 292, 17, 2105–14.

28 Weiss, G. *et al.*, 2002, 'Immunomodulation by perioperative administration of n-3 fatty acids', *Br J Nutr*, 87, Supp 1, S89–94.

29 Meydani, S.N. *et al.*, 1993, 'Immunologic effects of national cholesterol education panel step-2 diets with and without fish-derived n-3 fatty acid enrichment', *J Clin Invest*, 92, 105–13.

30 Simopoulos, A.P., 2002, 'Omega 3 fatty acids in inflammation and autoimmune diseases', *J Am College Nutrition*, 21, 495.

30 Miyao, M. *et al.*, 2000, 'Association of methylenetetrahydrofolate reductase (MTHFR) polymorphism with bone mineral density in postmenopausal Japanese women', *Calcif Tissue Int*, 66, 190–4.

31 Cauley, J.A. *et al.*, 1999, 'Apolipoprotein E polymorphism: a new genetic marker of hip fracture risk – the study of osteoporotic fractures', *J Bone Miner Res*, 14, 1175–81.

32 Frikke-Schimdt, R. *et al.*, 2000, 'Context-dependent and invariant associations between lipids, lipoproteins and apolipoproteins and apolipoprotein D genotype', *J Lipid Res*, 41, 11, 1812–22.

33 Corbo, R.M. *et al.*, 1999, 'Apolipoprotein (APOE) allele distribution in the world. Is APOE*4 a "thrifty" allele?', *Ann Hum Genet*, 63, 4, 301–10.

34 Kesaniemi, Y.A. *et al.*, 1987, 'Intestinal cholesterol absorption efficiency in man in related to apolipoprotein E phenotype', *J Clin Invest*, 80, 2, 578–81.

Chapter 9

1 Miekeley, N. 2001, 'Elemental anomalies in hair as indicators of endocrinologic pathologies and deficiencies in calcium and bone metabolism', *J Trace Elem Med Biol*, 15, 1, 46–55.

Chapter 10

1 Francis. R.M., 1997, 'Men and Bone – the rise in osteoporotic fractures', *Geriatric Medicine*, 31–7.

2 Amory, J.K., 2004, 'Exogenous testosterone or testosterone with finasteride increases bone mineral density in older men with low serum testosterone', *J Clin Endocrinol Metab*, 89, 503–10.

3 Deleat, C.E.D. *et al.*, 1997, 'Bone density and risk of hip fracture in men and women: cross-sectional analysis', *British Medical Journal*, 315, 221–5.

4 Tucker, K.L. *et al.*, 1999, 'Potassium and fruit and vegetables are associated with greater bone mineral density in elderly men and women', *American Journal of Clinical Nutrition*, 69, 727–36.

5   Hannan, M.T. *et al.*, 2000, 'Risk factors for longitudinal bone loss in elderly men and women: the Framingham Osteoporosis Study', *J Bone Miner Res*, 15, 710–20.

6   Dawson-Hughes, B. *et al.*, 1997, 'Effect of calcium and vitamin D supplementation on bone density in men and women 65 years of age or older', *New England Journal of Medicine*, 337, 670–6.

7   Dawson-Hughes, B. *et al.*, 2000, 'Effect of withdrawal of calcium and vitamin D supplements on bone mass in elderly men and women', *American Journal of Clinical Nutrition*, 72, 3, 745–50.

Chapter 11

1   Information taken from Remer, T. and Manz, F., 1995, 'Potential renal acid load of foods and its influence on urine pH', *J Am Diet Assoc*, 95, 791–7.

Index

Acknowledgements

There are a number of people I would like to thank as a lot goes on behind the scenes when writing a book. My thanks go to Louise Atkinson who helped to make this book more readable and stopped me from getting too technical.

Muna Reyal, my editor, has an eye like a hawk and can pick up errors miles away and my thanks go to her and everyone at Kyle Cathie for their help in publishing this book. I would like to say a special thanks and appreciation to Kyle whom I have worked with other the last eight years. I know people have horror stories about their publishers but I have only ever felt support and encouragement from her.

I would also like to give very special thanks to all the administrative team at my clinic in Tunbridge Wells (Mel, Brenda, Jenny, Jo, Trine, Len and Wendy) who have kept the clinics running smoothly while I shut myself away. They took a great weight off me which gave me time and space to really focus on this book with no other distractions. In particular, my thanks go to Alison Belcourt, who manages the nutrition department very expertly and who helped cover while I was away writing, and to Helen Heap who works with Alison.

Dr Michael Culp kindly read the genetics chapter and gave me some very useful comments. Julie Wallace was also really helpful with the recipes and I would like to thank her too. I know they always come last in the acknowledgements but they are no means least and I would like to send my love to my family, Kriss, Matt, Len and Chantell for all the emotional support and love they give me.